Radiation Therapy Study Guide

Amy Heath

Radiation Therapy Study Guide

A Radiation Therapist's Review

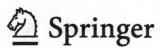

Amy Heath, MS, RT(T)
University of Wisconsin Hospital and Clinics
Madison, WI, USA

University of Wisconsin-LaCrosse
LaCrosse, WI, USA

ISBN 978-1-4939-3257-3   ISBN 978-1-4939-3258-0   (eBook)
DOI 10.1007/978-1-4939-3258-0

Library of Congress Control Number: 2015950844

Springer New York Heidelberg Dordrecht London

Printed on acid-free paper

Springer Science+Business Media LLC New York is part of Springer Science+Business Media
(www.springer.com)

Disclaimer

Though Amy Heath was an ARRT Item Writer, by binding contract, Amy Heath cannot reveal in whole or in part any of ARRT's copyrighted questions or any other insider information about the ARRT's examinations. The ARRT does not review, evaluate, or endorse review courses, activities, materials, or products and this disclaimer should not be construed as an endorsement by the ARRT.

Preface

This book is designed as a comprehensive review and study tool for radiation therapists to help them learn the many facets of radiation therapy. Organized in a question-and-answer format, with rationales for each answer provided, the material is geared towards the entry-level radiation therapist. Topics include radiation therapy physics, radiobiology, treatment and simulation equipment, principles of patient care, clinical components of cancer care, and individual chapters on cancers of the brain, head and neck region, and respiratory, digestive, urinary, and male and female reproductive systems. It is a valuable resource for radiation therapists preparing for certification examinations as well as for practicing therapists in need of a review.

As radiation therapists, we work in a field with cutting-edge technology. However, even with all of the changes in treatments and equipment, the exceptional care we provide to patients remains. Radiation therapy has been, and continues to be, a rewarding and fulfilling profession.

I hope that readers will find the material comprehensive and thought provoking.

Madison, WI, USA   Amy Heath, MS, RT(T)

Contents

Contents

Chapter 1
Radiation Physics

Questions

1. The orbital electron shell that is closest to the nucleus is:

    A. J
    B. K
    C. L
    D. M

2. The number of protons is an atom is also known as:

    A. Atomic mass number
    B. *A*
    C. Atomic number
    D. *X*

3. Isotopes have the same number of _____ and different number of _____.

    A. Neutrons, protons
    B. Electrons, neutrons
    C. Protons, neutrons
    D. Neutrons, electrons

4. With beta decay:

    A. Characteristic X-rays and Auger electrons are produced
    B. A positron and negatron are emitted from the nucleus
    C. A Helium nucleus is emitted
    D. A proton is transformed into a neutron

© Springer Science+Business Media New York 2016
A. Heath, *Radiation Therapy Study Guide*, DOI 10.1007/978-1-4939-3258-0_1

5. With electron capture (choose all correct answers):

   A. Characteristic X-rays and Auger electrons are produced
   B. Occurs in High Z materials
   C. A Helium nucleus is emitted
   D. A proton is transformed into a neutron

6. Which of the following radioisotopes is used for LDR GYN brachytherapy?

   A. I-131
   B. Cs-137
   C. Pd-103
   D. Ir-192

7. The half-life of Pd-103 is:

   A. 74.2 days
   B. 30 years
   C. 17 days
   D. 2.7 days

8. Which of the following is not a type of electromagnetic radiation?

   A. Microwaves
   B. Neutrons
   C. X-rays
   D. Radiowaves

9. Which of the following is true regarding the wavelength frequencies of electro-magnetic radiation?

   A. Wavelength is measured in hertz
   B. Wavelength and frequency are inversely related
   C. The product of frequency and wavelength is Planck's constant
   D. Frequency is represented by λ

10. When calculating attenuation with this formula, $I_x = I_0 e^{-\mu x}$, what does μ represent?

    A. Original intensity of the beam
    B. Thickness of the material the beam is passing through
    C. Linear attenuation coefficient of the material the beam is passing through
    D. Half-value layer of the material the beam is passing through

11. _____ describes the thickness of the medium needed to attenuate the beam's original intensity in half.

    A. Linear attenuation coefficient
    B. Half-value layer
    C. Inverse square law
    D. Decay constant

12. What term describes the relationship with beam intensity and distance from the source of a beam for photons as it travels through some medium?

    A. Linear attenuation coefficient
    B. Inverse square law
    C. Quantum model
    D. Transmission proportionality

13. Which of the following is not a filter used for low-energy treatment machines?

    A. Copper
    B. Thoraeus
    C. Tungston
    D. Aluminum

14. Which photon interaction with matter is most likely to occur with diagnostic imaging?

    A. Coherent scattering
    B. Photoelectric effect
    C. Compton effect
    D. Pair production
    E. Photodisintegration

15. Which photon interaction with matter is most likely to occur with radiation therapy delivery via linear accelerators?

    A. Coherent scattering
    B. Photoelectric effect
    C. Compton effect
    D. Pair production
    E. Photodisintegration

16. Which photon interaction with matter is most likely to occur with radiation therapy delivery via orthovoltage?

    A. Coherent scattering
    B. Photoelectric effect
    C. Compton effect
    D. Pair production
    E. Photodisintegration

17. What interaction is responsible for neutron contamination in radiation therapy?

    A. Coherent scattering
    B. Photoelectric effect
    C. Compton effect
    D. Pair production
    E. Photodisintegration

18. Pair production occurs in _____.

    A. Photon beams ≥ 1.022 keV
    B. Photon beams ≥ 1.022 MeV
    C. Electron beams ≥ 1.022 keV
    D. Electron beams ≥ 1.022 MeV

19. In the coherent scattering interaction, the energy of the ejected photon is _____ than the incident photon.

    A. Lower
    B. Greater
    C. Equal
    D. A photon is not ejected in coherent scattering

20. Which of the following is not true regarding inelastic electron-electron collisions?

    A. Occurs in matter with high Z
    B. Rate of energy loss is dependent on density of the matter it passes through
    C. Incident electrons do not interact with electrons of the matter in which it passes through
    D. Kinetic energy is not lost

21. The _____ tail is seen at the end of electron depth dose curves.

    A. Bragg
    B. Bremsstrahlung
    C. Characteristic
    D. Auger

22. Proton and alpha particles exhibit a _____ peak at the end of their range of travel, where most of their energy is deposited.

    A. Bragg
    B. Bremsstrahlung
    C. Characteristic
    D. Auger

23. What is not true regarding neutron interactions?

    A. Are directly ionizing
    B. Wax and water are used for blocking neutrons
    C. Interact with the nucleus
    D. Do not lose much energy when they react with target nuclei

24. The traditional unit for exposure is:

    A. Gray
    B. Roentgens (R)
    C. Rem
    D. Rad

25. Absorbed dose is measured in (choose all correct answers):

    A. Gray
    B. Becquerel
    C. Rem
    D. Rad
    E. Sievert

26. What is not true regarding dose equivalent?

    A. Rem is the SI unit
    B. Gamma rays have a QF of 1
    C. Alpha particles have a QF of 20
    D. Can be measured in Sv

27. Decay constant (λ) can be determined by dividing the element's half-life by:

    A. 10^{-3}
    B. 2.7×10^{11} Ci
    C. 0.693
    D. 100 ergs/g

28. Which of the following are used to calibrate linear accelerators?

    A. Pocket ionization chambers
    B. Cutie pie ionization chambers
    C. Thimble chambers
    D. Geiger-Muller chambers

29. Patient dose monitoring can be accurately measured with:

    A. Radiographic film
    B. Diode detectors
    C. Neutron detectors
    D. Farmer chambers

Answers and Rationales

1. B. Atoms, the smallest unit of mass, are made up of a nucleus (with neutrons and protons) of a positive charge, enclosed by orbital electrons. The K shell is closest to nucleus, then L, M, N, and O. The number of electrons in each shell can be quantified by $2n^2$, where n is the shell number.
2. C. Atomic number quantifies the number of protons in an atom (Z), while atomic mass number (A) quantifies the number of neutrons and protons in an atom.
3. C. Isotopes have the same number of protons and different number of neutrons. Isotones have the same number of neutrons and different number of protons. Isobars have the same mass number (protons + neutrons), but a different number of protons.
4. B. There are different modes of radioactive decay—alpha decay, beta decay, electron capture and gamma decay/isomeric transition. With alpha decay, two protons and two neutrons are emitted as a single alpha particle (helium nucleus). Alpha decay occurs in radionuclides with $Z>82$. Beta decay involves the ejection of a positive electron (positron) or negative electron (negatron) from the nucleus. Positrons are emitted during proton decay, and are accompanied by a neutrino. Negatrons are emitted during neutron decay, and are accompanied by an antineutrino. In electron capture, an orbital electron is captured by the nucleus, which transforms a proton into a neutron. Characteristic X-rays and Auger electrons are produced as electrons fall into orbital vacancies. Finally, with gamma decay/isomeric transition, a metastable nucleus undergoes nuclear decay, giving off gamma rays; this is always part of another decay process.
5. A and D. Please see Question 4 for details about radioactive decay.
6. B. See Table 1.1 for Radioisotopes, their uses and half-lives.
7. C. See Table 1.1 for Radioisotopes, their uses and half-lives.
8. B. Electromagnetic radiation is identified by alternating electric and magnetic fields, which are perpendicular to one another and the direction of their energy transmission. The electromagnetic spectrum includes X-rays, cosmic rays, UV lights, visible light, microwaves, and radiowaves. Electromagnetic radiation will interact with tissue by three ways: be absorbed by the medium, be scattered by the medium, travel through the medium with no interactions.
9. B. Wavelength (measured in meters) is the distance between peaks of waves. Frequency is measured by the number of oscillations/second or hertz.

Table 1.1 Commonly used radioisotopes

Radioisotope	Half-life	Clinical use
Iridium 192	74.2 days	HDR brachytherapy
Gold 198	2.7 days	Prostate seed implants
Cesium 137	30 years	LDR GYN brachytherapy
Palladium 103	17 days	Prostate seed implants
Iodine 125	60 days	Prostate seed implants

Wavelength and frequency are inversely related (i.e.: longer the wavelength the less the frequency); c (velocity)$=\nu$ (frequency)$\times\lambda$ (wavelength). Quantum model is also used to describe this relationship for photons; E (Energy in joules)$=h$ (Planck's constant)$\times\nu$.

10. C. Attenuation is the absorption or scatter of a radiation beam as it travels through a medium. The degree of attenuation can be calculated mathematically with the formula $I_x=I_0e^{-\mu x}$.

   - I_x: Intensity of the beam after passing through medium
   - I_0: Original intensity of the beam
   - μ: Linear attenuation coefficient of the medium and beam energy
   - x: Thickness of medium (in cm)

11. B. Half-value layer (HVL) describes the thickness of the medium needed to attenuate the beam's original intensity in half. HVL$=0.693/\mu$. The beam becomes harder as it travels through material, so the first HVL is less than the second and the second is less than the third, etc.

12. B. The intensity of the beam as it attenuates through a medium follows the inverse square law. For photons, beam intensity is inversely proportionate to the square of the distance from the source ($I_2=I_1(d_1/d_2)^2$).

13. C. Beam quality can be described by half-value layer (HVL), kVp and filtration. Filters are used to harden low energy photon beams. Aluminum filters are used for diagnostic photon beams. For orthovoltage, copper filters (1–4 mm) and Thoraeus filters are used. Thoraeus is made up of tin, copper and aluminum with tin being placed closest to the tube.

14. B. The photoelectric effect occurs in beams ≤ 1 MeV (primarily diagnostic radiology and orthovoltage) and is more likely to occur in matter which has a high Z. An incident photon interacts with inner shell electron, transferring all of its energy to the electron. The electron is then ejected and has an energy of the incident photon minus the binding energy of the electron. Characteristic X-rays are emitted as electrons from outer shells drop into the vacant orbits. Auger electrons may also be emitted.

15. C. The Compton effect occurs in beams 30 keV–30 MeV, and is independent of the atomic number of the medium it is passing through but is dependent on the electron density of the material. The incident photon interacts with outer shell electron, transferring some of its energy. This incident photon (now with less energy) changes direction and continues through. The electron (now with more energy) is emitted. The angles the photon and electron travel are dependent on the collision: direct hit (photon travels backward and electron travels forward), grazing hit (photon travels forward and electron travels at a right angle), and 90° scatter (photon is scattered at 90°, with the maximum energy of the photon$=0.511$ MeV).

16. B. The photoelectric effect occurs in beams ≤ 1 MeV (primarily diagnostic radiology and orthovoltage) and is more likely to occur in matter which has a high Z.

17. E. Photodisintegration occurs in photon beams ≥ 10 MeV, and occurs more often in mediums with a high atomic number (such as shielding material in

linear accelerators). In this interaction, an incident photon is completely absorbed by the nucleus of the target atom. Neutrons are emitted in order to create stability in the atom once again, which is responsible for neutron contamination in radiation therapy.

18. B. Pair production occurs in photon beams ≥1.022 MeV, and the probability of this reaction increases with energy and is dependent on the atomic number of the medium. An incident photon interacts with the electric field of the nucleus and converts its energy into two particles (an electron and positron). The positron will further interact with a free electron, undergoing an annihilation reaction which results in two photons of 0.511 MeV exiting in opposite directions.

19. C. Coherent scattering occurs in very low energy beams and high Z materials. The incident photon is low energy, so no ionization occurs. This incident photon energy is transferred to medium, which ejects a photon of the same energy as the incident photon. Coherent scattering is not experienced in radiation therapy.

20. B. Electrons lose energy as they pass through medium through ionizations and excitations. Different interactions include elastic (kinetic energy is not lost) and inelastic (some kinetic energy is lost through ionization or excitation). With inelastic electron-electron collisions, incident electrons can interact with electrons of the matter in which it passes through. The energy is given to the target electron (which can be ionized or excited) and the incident electron passes through (but now has less energy). Characteristic X-rays are produced if the target electron is ionized, as other electrons fill the empty spots in each shell. This type of collision is important in matter with low Z (water and tissue). The rate of energy loss is dependent on density of the matter it passes through; electrons ≥1 MeV in water lose energy at a rate of 2 MeV/cm.

21. B. The Bremsstrahlung tail at the end of electron depth dose curves represents the photon contamination created by inelastic electron-nuclei collisions. In this type of collision, incident electrons pass by the nucleus, are attracted its charge. It slows down by the nucleus (brakes) and changes direction. Kinetic energy is loss and emitted as a photon.

22. A. Charged particles such as electrons, protons, and alpha particles interact with medium by creating ionization and excitation. An incoming particle collides with the nucleus of the target, and loss of energy or bremsstrahlung reactions occur. Multiple scattering reactions by the incoming particles occur. Electrons scatter more than protons and alpha particles due to their small mass. Proton and alpha particles exhibit a Bragg peak at the end of their range of travel, where most of their energy is deposited.

23. A. Neutron interactions are indirectly ionizing. The neutrons interact with tissue by collisions with the target nucleus, which creates additional reactions in the cell, or nuclear disintegrations, which also causes additional reactions in the cell. Neutrons do not lose much energy when they react with target nuclei which are heavy. Therefore, water, wax, and polyethylene are useful materials for blocking neutrons.

24. B. Exposure is the amount of ionizations produced by photons per unit of mass in air. The SI unit for exposure is C/kg, while the traditional unit is Roentgens (R). $1\ R = 2.58 \times 10^{-4}$ C/kg.

25. A and D. Absorbed dose is defined as energy absorbed per unit mass. The SI unit for absorbed dose is the gray (Gy); $1\ Gy = 1$ J/kg. Rad (radiation absorbed dose) is an older unit for absorbed dose; $1\ rad = 100$ ergs/g. The relationship between Gy and rads is $100\ rad = 1$ Gy or $1\ rad = 1$ cGy. Becquerel (Bq) is the SI unit for radioactivity and is equal to 1 disintegrations per second (dps), which is equal to 2.7×10^{-11} Curies (Ci).

26. A. Dose equivalent is used to distinguish the different damage done to tissue by differing radiation. The SI unit for dose equivalent is Sievert (Sv); $1\ Sv = 1\ Gy \times$ Quality Factor (QF) of the radiation type. Rem is the traditional unit; $1\ rem = 1\ rad \times QF$. X-rays, gamma rays, electrons, beta particles, and some protons have a QF of 1, while thermal neutrons have a QF of 5, and fast neutrons and alpha particles have a QF of 20.

27. C. Activity describes the rate of decay of an element. Activity can be calculated by $A = A_0 e^{-\lambda t}$.

   - A = Activity at time
   - A_0 = Activity at start of time
   - λ = decay constant; λ is related to the element's half-life ($T_{\frac{1}{2}} = 0.693/\lambda$)
   - t = time in seconds

28. C. Gas-filled ionization detectors include ionization chambers and Geiger-Muller chambers. Pocket ionization chambers can be used for personnel monitoring. Cutie pie chamber is a portable ionization chamber. Thimble chambers (including Farmer chambers) can be used for linear accelerator calibration. Geiger-Muller chambers are more sensitive than ionization chambers, thus are frequently used for detecting low levels of radiation. While they cannot measure dose, they can be used to detect radiation (useful for finding lost sources or radiation surveys).

29. B. Diode detectors measure dose and dose rate (for photons and electrons) and are often used for patient dose monitoring due to small size and instant reading. Radiographic film may be used to verify portals. Silver bromide crystals produce a latent image on film once irradiated. After processing, the optical density of the film is proportional to the amount of radiation exposure. Neutron detectors are ionization chambers filled with BF_3 gas to detect and measure neutrons for radiation protection areas.

Suggested Readings

Blinick JS, Quate EG. Radiation safety and protection. In: Washington CM, Leaver D, editors. Principles and practice of radiation therapy. 3rd ed. St. Louis, MO: Mosby Elsevier; 2010. p. 347–62.

Hendee WR, Ibbott GS, Hendee EG. Radiation therapy physics. 3rd ed. Hoboken, NJ: Wiley; 2005.

Khan FM. The physics of radiation therapy. 4th ed. Baltimore, MD: Lippincott Williams & Wilkins; 2010.

Leaver D, Miller AC. Medical imaging. In: Washington CM, Leaver D, editors. Principles and practice of radiation therapy. 3rd ed. St. Louis, MO: Mosby Elsevier; 2010. p. 103–32.

Sahoo N. Introduction to radiation therapy physics. In: Washington CM, Leaver D, editors. Principles and practice of radiation therapy. 3rd ed. St. Louis, MO: Mosby Elsevier; 2010. p. 277–99.

Stanton R, Stinson D. Applied physics for radiation oncology. Madison, WI: Medical Physics Publishing; 1996.

Chapter 2
Radiation Protection and Safety

Questions

1. What acronym represents the fundamental radiation safety principle used in radiation therapy?

   A. ALARA
   B. OAR
   C. DVH
   D. HVL

2. The three principles of ALARA include:

   A. Personnel and facilities monitoring
   B. Time
   C. Neutron contamination
   D. Distance
   E. Shielding

3. Regarding radiation protection for photon beams, which of the following would have the greatest effect to minimize dose?

   A. Double the shielding
   B. Double the time
   C. Double the distance
   D. All of the above would have an equal effect

4. What organization sets the recommended dose limits for radiation workers and the general public?

   A. NRC
   B. NCRP
   C. ACR
   D. ASRT

© Springer Science+Business Media New York 2016
A. Heath, *Radiation Therapy Study Guide*, DOI 10.1007/978-1-4939-3258-0_2

5. The annual dose equivalent limit for whole-body occupational exposure is:

   A. 0.05 rem
   B. 0.5 rem
   C. 5 rem
   D. 50 rem

6. The annual dose equivalent limit for occupational exposure of the extremity is:

   A. 0.05 rem
   B. 0.5 rem
   C. 5 rem
   D. 50 rem

7. Personnel must be monitored for radiation exposure if they are expected to receive ___% of the dose equivalent limit.

   A. 10
   B. 30
   C. 50
   D. 70

8. What is not an advantage of the use of film badge dosimeters for personnel monitoring?

   A. Inexpensive
   B. Can be used for different types and energies of radiation
   C. Easy to use
   D. Accurate

9. Thermoluminescent dosimeters are commonly made of what material?

   A. Lithium fluoride
   B. Aluminum oxide
   C. Silver bromide
   D. Sulfur hexafluoride

10. Which of the following personnel monitors provides immediate readings?

   A. Film badge dosimeters
   B. Thermoluminescent dosimeters
   C. Optically stimulated luminescence dosimeter
   D. Pocket ionization chambers

11. What is an advantage of using optically stimulated luminescence dosimeter (OSL) over another type of personnel dosimeter?

   A. Can be read immediately
   B. Can detect different energies of radiation
   C. Are the most inexpensive personnel dosimeter
   D. Do not require additional equipment to measure readings

12. Caution—Radiation Area signs are used to identify areas in which radiation workers may receive:

   A. Any amount of radiation
   B. 5 mrem/h
   C. 100 mrem/h
   D. 500 mrem/h

13. Which of the following is not true regarding radiation protection surveys?

   A. Geiger-Muller counters are used to measure exposure
   B. Are used to verify exposure levels
   C. Completed periodically per regulatory body recommendations
   D. Are used to ensure shielding levels are adequate

14. When determining shielding of radiation oncology departments, work load describes:

   A. How often the beam is on each week
   B. Fraction of time beam is directed at each barrier
   C. Fraction of time the adjacent area will be occupied
   D. Distance from source of radiation to adjacent area

15. An occupancy factor of _____ should be used for control rooms when planning shielding thickness.

   A. 50
   B. ½
   C. 1
   D. 100

Answers and Rationales

1. A. ALARA (As Low As Reasonably Achievable) is the fundamental radiation safety principle—the lower the dose received, the lower the risk of the individual irradiated.

2. B, D, and E. For external beam exposure, ALARA can be achieved by following the rules of time, distance, and shielding.

3. C. Time has a direct relationship, so the less time exposed, the less dose received. Distance, on the other hand, has an indirect relationship—increasing distance from radiation source, decreases dose. In this instance, the Inverse Square Law applies (i.e.: double the distance, decrease dose received by 4). Finally, shielding should be maximized. Lead, concrete and steel are used for megavoltage equipment, and the thickness required depends on type and energy of radiation. Shielding required is specified by half-value layers (HVL), or the thickness of material needed to reduce the intensity to one-half of the original value or tenth-value layer (TVL), or the thickness of material needed to reduce the intensity to one-tenth of the original value.

4. B. National Council on Radiation Protection and Measurement (NCRP) sets recommended dose limits for radiation workers and the general public. Limits are outlined in NCRP Report No 116. The recommended limits are higher for radiation workers than the general public.

5. C

6. D. See Table 2.1 for recommended dose limits. Limits do not include doses from background or medical procedures.

7. A. Personnel must be monitored for exposure if expected to receive 10 % of the dose equivalent limit. Personnel monitoring is useful for determining the amount of radiation exposure an occupational worker received in a given period of time, allows the facility and radiation safety officer to determine any safety concerns, and serves as a permanent record an occupational worker received.

Table 2.1 NCRP recommendations for dose limits

Occupational exposure, whole body (annual)	5 rem
Occupational exposure, lens eye	15 rem
Occupational exposure, other tissues and organs	50 rem
Occupational exposure, cumulative dose	1 rem × age in years
Public dose limit, infrequent exposure	0.5 rem
Embryo-fetus exposure (total limit)	0.5 rem
Embryo-fetus exposure (per month limit)	0.05 rem

Source: Blinick and Quate (2010), Khan (2010), Meihold et al. (1993)

Whole body monitors are worn on chest or abdomen; ring badges are worn if high dose to that area is expected.

8. D. Film badge dosimeters are worn by radiation workers, and the optical densities of the film are then measured to determine exposure. While film badge dosimeters are inexpensive and easy to use, and can discern doses between different energies of radiation through the use of filters, they can be inaccurate. The film should not be exposed to heat or humidity and the badges cannot be read immediately.

9. A. Thermoluminescent dosimeters (TLD) are commonly made of lithium fluoride and are most often used in ring badges. A fraction of the absorbed energy is caught in the lattice work of the crystal component of the dosimeter after irradiated. This energy is released as light when the dosimeter is heated at a later time, and the amount of light is proportional to radiation exposure. TLDs are more precise than film badge dosimeters, and not as sensitive to heat and humidity as film. However, they cannot determine energy of radiation received, are expensive, and cannot be read immediately.

10. D. Pocket ionization chambers (pocket dosimeters) are pen sized ionization chambers that can be read at any time. They can be read immediately, and be used over and over, but the up-front cost for these devices is high. In addition, the readings can be inaccurate if exposed to humidity or mechanical shock.

11. B. When OSLs are irradiated, electrons are trapped in aluminum oxide, which give off light when exposed to lasers. The amount of light is proportional to radiation exposure. This type of personnel dosimeter is very sensitive, can be read multiple times, and with the use of filters, can accurately detect different energies of radiation. However, they cannot be read immediately.

12. B. In a controlled radiation area, the following signs may be used (Table 2.2).

13. A. Radiation surveys should be completed for all areas in and around a radiation area to verify exposure levels and ensure shielding is adequate. The surveys are completed initially, and periodically thereafter dependent on regulatory bodies' recommendations. Radiation surveys are completed with ionization chambers (Cutie pie) to measure exposure, or Geiger-Muller counters to determine the presence of radiation.

14. A. Factors to determine shielding include Workload (W): how often the beam is on each week; dependent on number of patients and radiation dose to each,

Table 2.2 Radiation warning signs

Caution—Radioactive Material	Sign used to identify where radioactive material is present (i.e., cesium bank, radioactive packages)
Caution—Radiation Area	Sign used to identify areas in which radiation workers may receive >5 mrem/h
Caution—High Radiation Area	Sign used to identify areas in which the dose rate >100 mrem/h
Caution—Grave Danger, Very High Radiation Area	Sign used to identify areas in which the dose rate >500 cGy/h

Use factor (U): fraction of time beam is directed at each barrier, Occupancy factor (T): fraction of time the adjacent area will be occupied, Distance (d): distance from source of radiation to adjacent area and Effective dose equivalent limit for occupied area (P): public or occupational. Shielding designed to block the useful beam is the primary barrier [B (required transmission factor) $=(P \times d^2)/WUT$]. Shielding designed to block leakage and scatter radiation is the secondary barrier. Shielding is not designed to block background radiation.

15. C. Occupancy factors are as follows: Full occupancy: $T = 1$ (control rooms and offices), Partial occupancy: $T = 1/4$ (hallways and restrooms), Occasional occupancy: $T = 1/8 - 1/16$ (closets and stairwells).

Suggested Readings

Blinick JS, Quate EG. Radiation safety and protection. In: Washington CM, Leaver D, editors. Principles and practice of radiation therapy. 3rd ed. St. Louis, MO: Mosby Elsevier; 2010. p. 347–62.

Hendee WR, Ibbott GS, Hendee EG. Radiation therapy physics. 3rd ed. Hoboken, NJ: Wiley; 2005.

Khan FM. The physics of radiation therapy. 4th ed. Baltimore, MD: Lippincott Williams & Wilkins; 2010.

Meihold CB, Abrahamson S, Adelstein SJ, Bair WJ, Boice JD, Fry RJM, et al. Limitation of exposure to ionizing radiation. Bethesda, MD: National Council on Radiation Protection & Measurements; 1993. Report No.: 116.

Stanton R, Stinson D. Applied physics for radiation oncology. Madison, WI: Medical Physics Publishing; 1996.

Chapter 3
Radiobiology

Questions

1. Which is true regarding direct effects of radiation?

   A. Occurs more often with low LET radiation
   B. Occurs more often with high LET radiation
   C. Interacts with the water in the cell
   D. Increases with an increase in oxygen

2. Which is true regarding indirect effects of radiation?

   A. Cannot be modified by chemical factors
   B. Target is the DNA of the cell
   C. Occurs with neutrons
   D. More common with high LET radiation

3. Which of the following is not an example of chromosome damage resulting from ionizing radiation?

   A. Double-strand break
   B. Translocation
   C. Ring formation
   D. Anaphase bridge

4. What cellular response to radiation is characterized by cells pausing in G2 to repair themselves prior to entering mitosis?

   A. Division delay
   B. Interphase death
   C. Reproductive failure
   D. DNA cross-linking

5. Acute effects are seen within _____ months of radiation exposure.

   A. 2
   B. 4
   C. 6
   D. 8

6. Which of the following is not true regarding non-stochastic late effects?

   A. Occur after a threshold dose is passed
   B. Severity of effect is proportionate to dose
   C. Probability of effect occurring is proportionate to dose
   D. Also referred to as a deterministic effect

7. Somatic effects of radiation:

   A. Occurs in the irradiated individual
   B. Is passed on to future generations
   C. Has a threshold dose
   D. Severity increases with increased dose

8. What is the definition of LD 50/30?

   A. Dose that will result in death in 50 % of individuals within 30 days
   B. Dose that will result in complications in 5 % of the population in 5 years
   C. Dose that will result in complications in 50 % of the population in 5 years
   D. Dose that will result in death in 50 % of individuals within 30 years

9. What is the TD 5/5 of the parotid gland?

   A. 17.5 Gy
   B. 23 Gy
   C. 32 Gy
   D. 55 Gy

10. What is the TD 5/5 of the brain?

   A. 30 Gy
   B. 35 Gy
   C. 40 Gy
   D. 45 Gy

11. What is the TD 5/5 of the bladder?

   A. 55 Gy
   B. 60 Gy
   C. 65 Gy
   D. 70 Gy

12. Exceeding the TD 5/5 of the lens will result in:

    A. Blindness
    B. Cataracts
    C. Retinal detachment
    D. Necrosis

13. After acute whole-body exposure, in what stage will the individual be relatively symptom free?

    A. Prodromal
    B. Latent
    C. Manifest illness
    D. In all stages some symptoms will be experienced

14. What is true regarding the hematopoietic syndrome following acute whole-body radiation exposure?

    A. Occurs in doses between 20 and 30 Gy
    B. Manifest illness occurs 3–5 days after exposure
    C. Effects may be reversed with bone marrow transplant or protective isolation
    D. Mucosal layer of the small bowel is damaged

15. An acute dose of 40 Gy would result in death in:

    A. Hours
    B. 2 days
    C. 10 days
    D. 30 days

16. Which is not true regarding cerebrovascular syndrome following acute whole-body exposure?

    A. Occurs in doses >50 Gy
    B. Prodromal and latent period may be nonexistent
    C. Manifest illness occurs within hours of exposure, marked by convulsions and coma
    D. Death occurs within 3 h

17. Which of the following is an effect of radiation to the fetus?

    A. Lethal effect
    B. Malformations
    C. Growth retardation
    D. All are effects

18. Dose limits for a fetus of a radiation worker who has declared their pregnancy is:

    A. 0.5 mSv/term
    B. 5 mSv/term
    C. 0.5 mSv/month
    D. 5 mSv/month

19. Radiosensitivity of a cell increases with:

    A. Decreased mitotic activity
    B. Increased specialization
    C. Increased mitotic activity
    D. Decreased oxygen within the cell

20. The most radiosensitive phase of the cell cycle is:

    A. G1
    B. S
    C. G2
    D. M

21. The most important radiosensitizer is:

    A. WR 2721
    B. Carbotaxol
    C. Oxygen
    D. Nitrogen

22. A known radioprotector is:

    A. WR 2721
    B. Carbotaxol
    C. Oxygen
    D. Nitrogen

23. What is true regarding the use of oxygen with radiation exposure?

    A. Oxygen has the greatest effect when administered prior to radiation exposure
    B. Oxygen has more of an effect with low LET
    C. Oxygen has the greatest effect when administered after radiation exposure
    D. Oxygen has minimal effect on the response of tissue to radiation

24. Linear Energy Transfer (LET) is measured in units of:

    A. keV/μm
    B. MeV/μm
    C. keV/mm
    D. MeV/mm

25. What is not true regarding relative biological effectiveness (RBE)?

    A. 250 MV is the control radiation used
    B. RBE increases with increased LET
    C. RBE increases with increased OER
    D. RBE compares different types of radiation

26. Liver cells fall into what category, specific to their radiosensitivity?

    A. Vegetative intermitotic cells (VIM)
    B. Differentiating intermitotic cells (DIM)
    C. Reverting postmitotic cells (RPM)
    D. Fixed postmitotic cells (FPM)

27. The cell survival curves used in radiation therapy are described as:

    A. Linear-exponential model
    B. Alpha-linear model
    C. Single target, multi-hit model
    D. Linear-quadratic model

28. In a cell survival curve, Dq represents:

    A. Width of the shoulder of the cell survival curve
    B. Extrapolation number
    C. Dose at which 63 % of cells are killed
    D. Dose at which 37 % of cells are killed

29. For mammalian cells, what is the typical range for "n" in the cell survival curve?

    A. −10 to 2
    B. 2–10
    C. 12–20
    D. 18–25

30. Protraction describes:

    A. Dividing the total dose into multiple fractions to improve tumor control and reduce normal effects
    B. The time in which the total dose is delivered
    C. The total dose the patient receives
    D. Increased dose per fraction with decreased number of fractions

31. Which of the four Rs of radiobiology describes the fixing of sublethal damage?

    A. Repair
    B. Repopulation
    C. Redistribution
    D. Reoxygenation

32. The alpha-beta ratio for early effects is:

    A. 3 Gy
    B. 6 Gy
    C. 10 Gy
    D. 14 Gy

33. Hypofractionation uses:

    A. Multiple fractions per day
    B. Lower dose per fraction
    C. Increased number of fractions
    D. Increased dose per fraction

34. Which is not true regarding hyperfractionation:

    A. Goal is to decrease late effects in normal tissue
    B. Fractions should be delivered 3 h apart
    C. Treated with lower dose per fraction
    D. Total dose is increased

Answers and Rationales

1. B. Direct effects of radiation cause damage directly to DNA and is more common high linear energy transfer (LET) radiation. Direct radiation effects occur with charged particles (alpha particles, protons, electrons) and cannot be modified by physical, biological, and chemical factors.
2. C. Indirect effects of radiation react with water, causing free radicals to form which eventually causes damage to DNA. While more common with low LET radiation (X-rays and gamma rays), it also occurs with neutrons and can be modified by physical, biological and chemical factors.
3. A. Ionizing radiation can cause chromosome damage and DNA damage. Types of chromosome damage include inversions and deletions, translocations, dicentric formation, ring formation, and anaphase bridge. DNA damage include double-strand breaks, single-strand breaks, change in base sequence, and cross-linking within the DNA.
4. A. Cellular response to radiation varies. Cells may experience no response. Division delay may also occur, in which cells pause in G2 to repair themselves before entering mitosis. In interphase death, cells die before mitosis (in G1, S, or G2 phase). Interphase death is more likely to occur in cells that do not actively divide (nerves), as well as cells that rapidly proliferate (lymphocytes). With reproductive failure, cells lose their ability to divide after radiation exposure and die in mitosis, or undergo apoptosis.
5. C. Radiation response is dependent on dose received, volume irradiated, and reparability of the structure. Acute effects are seen within 6 months of exposure, while late effects are seen after 6 months of exposure.
6. C. Non-stochastic late effects are those that occur after a threshold dose is passed, such as radiation myelitis, and is also referred to as a deterministic effect. With non-stochastic late effects, the severity of effect is proportionate to dose (once threshold is met). Threshold doses and late sequelae have been summarized by Emami (TD 5/5s) and QUANTEC (Quantitative Analysis of Normal Tissue Effects in Clinic). With stochastic late effects, any exposure can induce effect and an increased dose results in increase probability that the effect will occur, but does not increase the severity of the effect.
7. A. Somatic effects occur in the individual irradiated, such as carcinogenesis. Leukemia can occur 4–7 years after exposure, while solid tumors can occur 10–20 years after exposure. Genetic effects are passed on to future generations. Both somatic and genetic effects are stochastic late effects of radiation.
8. A. The LD 50/30 is the dose that will result in death in 50 % of individuals within 30 days, and is ~3 Gy, though difficult to specify due to lack of data in humans. TD 5/5 is the dose that will result in complications in 5 % of the population in 5 years and the TD 50/5 is the dose that will result in complications in 50 % of the population in 5 years.
9. C
10. D

Table 3.1 TD 5/5 values

Organ	TD 5/5 for whole organ (Gy)	Outcome
Kidney	23	Nephritis
Brain	45	Necrosis
Brain stem	50	Infarction/necrosis
Optic nerve	50	Blindness
Optic chiasm	50	Blindness
Lens	10	Blindness
Retina	45	Blindness
Lung	17.5	Pneumonitis
Spinal cord	47	Myelitis/necrosis
Liver	30	Liver failure
Bladder	65	Contracture
Heart	40	Pericarditis
Esophagus	55	Ulceration/stricture
Stomach	50	Ulceration/perforation
Small intestine	40	Obstruction/perforation
Colon	45	Obstruction/perforation
Rectum	60	Ulceration/stricture
Parotid gland	32	Xerostomia
Skin per 100 cm^2	50	Necrosis/ulceration
Mandible	60	Necrosis
Thyroid	45	Reduced hormone production
Pituitary	45	Reduced hormone production
Larynx	45	Laryngeal edema
Larynx	70	Cartilage necrosis

Source: Emami B, et al.: Tolerance of normal tissue to therapeutic radiation. Int. J. Radiat. Oncol. Biol. Phys. 21: 109–122. 1991

11. C
12. B. See Table 3.1 for selected TD 5/5s and clinical endpoints.
13. B. Regardless of dose, individuals irradiated to the whole body in an acute expo-sure will experience reaction in three stages. The prodromal stage occurs right after exposure. Common side effects include nausea, vomiting, and other gastro-intestinal side effects. In the latent stage, the individual is relatively symptom free. During the manifest illness, the individual exhibits side effects of exposure.
14. C. The hematopoietic syndrome occurs in doses 1–10 Gy. The bone marrow is damaged and stem cells are depleted. Manifest illness occurs 3–5 weeks after exposure, marked by anemia and infection. Death occurs in weeks, though effects may be reversed with bone marrow transplant or protective isolation
15. C. The gastrointestinal syndrome occurs in doses 10–50 Gy, in which the muco-sal layer of small bowel is damaged. Manifest illness occurs within 5–10 days of exposure, marked by nausea and vomiting, diarrhea and fever and death occurs within 3–10 days.

16. D. The cerebrovascular syndrome occurs in doses >50 Gy. Prodromal and latent period may be nonexistent. Manifest illness occurs within hours of exposure, marked by convulsions and coma and death occurs within 3 days.

17. D. When an embryo and/or fetus are exposed to irradiation, the following effects may occur: lethal effect (more common when exposure occurs before or right after implantation), malformations (common when exposure occurs during organogenesis), and growth retardation (can occur when exposure occurs at any part of development, but is more prevalent with exposure during late pregnancy).

18. C. Radiation workers must declare their pregnancy in writing to their radiation safety officer to trigger fetal dose monitoring. Once pregnancy is declared, the maximum permissible dose is 0.5 mSv/month to fetus.

19. C. Law of Bergonie and Tribondeau states that cells with these characteristics are more sensitive to radiation: increased mitotic index, undifferentiated cells (stem cells), and long mitotic future (will go through many divisions).

20. D

21. C. Ancel and Vitemberger report cells are equally sensitive to radiation, but show their radiation damage if and when they divide. Cells that divide more often will appear more radiosensitive. Effect of radiation in cells can be modified by different factors: biological (cell cycle, repair of sublethal damage), chemical (radiosensitizers and radioprotectors), and physical (LET and RBE). Oxygen is the most important radiatiosensitizer.

22. A. Radioprotectors decrease cellular response to radiation. WR 2721 (Amofositine) is an example.

23. B. Oxygen enhancement ration (OER) describes response of cells to radiation with and without the presence of oxygen. Oxygen has the greatest effect when oxygen is present during radiation.

24. A. LET is energy transferred per unit length (keV/μm).

25. A. Relative biological effectiveness (RBE) compares different types of radiation in regards to a specific biological effect. A control radiation of 250 kvP beam is used. RBE increases with increased LET and OER (but increased LET has opposite effect on OER)

26. C. Rubin and Casarett grouped cells into categories based on their radiosensitivity. Vegetative intermitotic cells (VIM) divide rapidly and regularly, are undifferentiated and are the most radiosensitive group. Examples of VIM cells include basal cells and erythroblasts. Differentiating intermitotic cells (DIM), divide, but not as often as VIM cells and are more differentiated than VIM cells. Examples of DIM cells include spermatagonia and myelocytes. Multipotential connective tissue cells divide irregularly and somewhat radiosensitive. Examples include fibroblasts and endothelial cells. Reverting postmitotic cells (RPM) do not divide, but can if needed, and are radioresistant. Fixed postmitotic cells (FPM) do not divide, and are very specialized cells and the most radioresistant group. Examples of FPM cells include nerve and muscle cells.

27. D. Cell survival curves are a graphical display of cellular response to radiation, and show cells usually have more than one target (known as multitarget single hit model). Is a linear-quadratic model, as there are two components of cell killing.

One component is proportionate to dose (alpha) and the other component is proportionate to square of dose (beta). Alpha-beta ratio is the point where cell kill from each component is equal.

28. A. Dq is the quasithreshold dose, and measures width of shoulder. Dq can be found by drawing horizontal line across from 1 on y-axis until it meets the cell survival curve. Dq represents doses at which cells are repairing sublethal damage. High LET curves have no shoulder, because no sublethal damage occurs with this type of radiation. D_0 is the dose at which there is 63 % cell kill (or 37 % surviving fraction), and is the reciprocal of the slope of the linear portion of curve. The typical range of D_0 is 1–2 Gy for mammalian cells.

29. B. The extrapolation number or target number, n, is found by extrapolating the cell survival curve until it intersects with the y-axis. n represents the number of targets in cell and is typically between 2 and 10 for mammalian cells.

30. B. Fractionation is dividing the total dose into multiple fractions to improve tumor control and reduce normal effects, while protraction is the time in which the total dose is delivered.

31. A. Fractionation utilizes the four R's of radiobiology: repair of sublethal damage, repopulation (normal cells repopulate between fractions), redistribution or reassortment (cells are redistributed to other parts of the cell cycle), and reoxygenation (cells become more oxygenated and more sensitive).

32. C. Prolonging overall treatment time does not affect late reactions, but does decrease early reactions. Response to fraction size in regards to late effects is dependent on the cell's alpha-beta ratio. Alpha-beta ratio is 10 Gy for early effects and 3 Gy for late effects. Late responding tissues are more sensitive to fraction size.

33. D. Conventional fractionation is 180–200 cGy/day for 6–8 weeks. Hypofractionation uses an increased dose per fraction with decreased number of fractions, used in prostate cancer.

34. B. Hyperfractionation delivers a decreased dose per fraction, given more than once a day, with same overall treatment time and increased total dose. Hyperfractionation decreases late effects and has been shown to improve local control in head and neck cancer. Fractions should be delivered with 6 h between to allow sublethal repair of normal tissues.

Suggested Readings

Hall EJ, Giaccia AJ. Radiobiology for the radiologist. 7th ed. Philadelphia, PA: Lippincott Williams & Williams; 2012.

Vonkadich AC. Overview of radiobiology. In: Washington CM, Leaver D, editors. Principles and practice of radiation therapy. 3rd ed. St. Louis, MO: Mosby Elsevier; 2010. p. 57–85.

Chapter 4
Treatment and Simulation Equipment

Questions

1. The Dmax of a 10 MV photon beam is:

   A. 0.5 cm
   B. 1.0 cm
   C. 2.0 cm
   D. 2.5 cm

2. The source for microwave power in a LINAC with energies greater than 12 MeV is:

   A. Magnetron
   B. RF driver
   C. Klystron
   D. Circulating pump

3. In a LINAC, what structure transports the microwaves from the stand to the Accelerator Structure?

   A. Klystron
   B. Accelerating waveguide
   C. Bending magnet
   D. Waveguide

4. The cathode of the linear accelerator is the:

   A. Magnetron
   B. Electron gun
   C. Tungston target
   D. Bending magnet

© Springer Science+Business Media New York 2016
A. Heath, *Radiation Therapy Study Guide*, DOI 10.1007/978-1-4939-3258-0_4

5. What is not true regarding the accelerator structure of a linear accelerator?

   A. It is located in the stand of the linear accelerator
   B. They may be mounted vertically
   C. They may be mounted horizontally
   D. Electrons are accelerated in this component

6. Targets in a linear accelerator are typically made of:

   A. Tungsten
   B. Lead
   C. Copper
   D. Concrete

7. What is the average energy of a 15 MV photon beam?

   A. 3.75 MV
   B. 5 MV
   C. 7.5 MV
   D. 15 MV

8. The _____ sets the beam's maximum field size.

   A. Target
   B. Bending magnet
   C. Independent jaws
   D. Primary collimator

9. Which of the following components are in the beam for X-ray production in a LINAC? (Choose all correct answers).

   A. Scattering foil
   B. Target
   C. Flattening filter

10. What is moved out of the beam's path when treating with electrons? (Choose all correct answers).

    A. Target
    B. Scattering foil
    C. Flattening filter

11. What component of the linear accelerator is responsible for signaling the machine to shut off once the requested dose has been delivered?

    A. Pulsed power supply
    B. Ionization chamber
    C. Klystron
    D. Circulator

12. What are the collimator jaws of the linear accelerator?

    A. Primary collimators
    B. Secondary collimators
    C. Multileaf collimators
    D. None of the above

13. What component in the treatment head of the linear accelerator displays the SSD on the patient's skin?

    A. Field-defining light
    B. Optical distance indicator
    C. Electron applicator
    D. Mechanical distance indicator

14. The LINAC is pressurized with _____ to decrease a chance for electrical breakdown.

    A. Oil
    B. SF_6
    C. Radiofrequency
    D. Microwaves

15. What auxiliary system in the linear accelerator allows for changing the dose rate at the treatment console?

    A. Cooling system
    B. Vacuum system
    C. Automatic frequency control
    D. Pulsed power supply

16. Treatment couches are typically constructed of:

    A. Carbon fiber
    B. Lucite
    C. Lead
    D. Styrofoam

17. Which of the following is not an example of an on-board imaging device used for target localization?

    A. EPIDs
    B. KV Cone-Beam CT
    C. CT scanner on rails
    D. In room PET scanner

18. The X-ray tube of a conventional simulator is located in the:

    A. Stand
    B. Gantry
    C. Image intensifier
    D. Modulator cabinet

19. _____ depict the field size in a conventional simulator.

    A. Primary collimator
    B. Blades
    C. Wires
    D. Shutters

20. What part of the CT simulator is often referred to as the "bore"?

    A. X-ray tube
    B. Gantry
    C. Fan beam detectors
    D. X-ray tube

21. The Hounsfield unit of air is:

    A. +1000
    B. −1000
    C. 0
    D. −100

22. DRR stands for:

    A. Digitally reconstructed radiograph
    B. Digitally represented radiograph
    C. Diagnostic radiograph reconstruction
    D. Dose ratio reconstruction

23. Voxels represent the_____ of a CT image.

    A. Brightness
    B. Contrast
    C. Slice thickness
    D. Number of pixels

24. What advanced treatment delivery equipment is a LINAC mounted on a robotic arm?

    A. Tomotherapy
    B. Cyberknife
    C. Gamma knife
    D. Proton beam therapy

Answers and Rationales

1. D. Higher energy photons penetrate deeper in the body, and are more forward scattering. Dmax, or depth at which 100 % of dose is deposited, differs per different energies. Electronic equilibrium occurs here (Table 4.1).
2. C. The magnetron and klystron are located in the stand of the linear accelerator. A magnetron produces microwaves, and is less expensive and less stable than klystron. The klystron amplifies microwaves, and is used rather than magnetron in higher energy LINACS (>12 MeV).
3. D. Microwaves travel to gantry through waveguide. These copper pipes that contain microwaves, which are reflected off the walls. The circulator prevents backflow of microwaves into magnetron/klystron.
4. B. An electron gun (cathode of the LINAC) injects electrons into the accelerator structure. The electrons "ride" the microwave and are accelerated and bunched along the course of the accelerator structure.
5. A. Located in the gantry, accelerator structures are classified as traveling wave or standing wave (more common). Depending on the length of the accelerator structure, they may be mounted vertically (short length) or horizontally (long length). Microwaves meet electrons and are accelerated here.
6. A. If X-rays are needed for treatment, the electron beam hits a tungsten (or a similar high Z material) target, which is the anode of the LINAC.
7. B. The maximum energy of the X-ray beam is that of the incident electron beam energy. The average energy of the X-ray beam is approximately 1/3 of the incident electron beam energy.
8. D. The primary collimator helps shape the beam and sets the maximum field size, usually 40×40 cm.
9. B and C.
10. A and C. When treating with electron beams, the target is moved out the beam's path. After passing through the primary collimator, the beam strikes a scattering foil. Flattening filters are used for X-ray beams. After hitting the target, the intensity of the X-ray beam is primarily at the center of the beam. The metal flattening filter is thicker in the center and creates uniformity across the X-ray beam. Scattering foils are used for electron beams. The electron beam has a very small diameter and the scattering foils spread out the thin pencil beam into a useful beam for treatment.
11. B. After passing through the flattening filter or scattering foil, the beam next travels through an ionization chamber, which monitors dose rate and integrated

Table 4.1 Photon energies and corresponding Dmax depths

Photon energy (MV)	Depth of Dmax (cm)
4	1
6	1.5
10	2.5
18	3.5

dose. The ionization chamber is responsible for shutting machine off when desired dose is delivered.

12. B. Secondary collimators, or collimator jaws, are tungsten or lead jaws which set the field size for treatment. X jaws set width of field, and Y jaws set length of field. Modern LINACs are equipped with independent jaws for asymmetric fields.

13. B. The field defining light displays the light field which imitates radiation field, while the optical distance indicator displays SSD on patient's skin, and typically reads 80–130 cm. Electron applicator cones are available in multiple sizes, and attach to the machine with the accessory mount. They further define the beam and field shape when treating with electrons.

14. B. The pressure system of a linear accelerator uses SF_6 to pressurize waveguide, which decreases chance for electrical breakdown. SF_6 can break down into a toxic substance, so use care when the equipment has a gas fault.

15. D. The cooling system, located in the stand, uses temperature controlled water to dissipate heat of the LINAC. The vacuum system keeps low, constant pressure for the electron gun, accelerator structure, and bending magnet. The automatic frequency control keeps the frequency of LINAC running at optimal level. The pulsed power supply is located in a detached modular cabinet and provides energy to klystron and electron gun and allows for changing the dose rate.

16. A. The treatment couch is made of carbon fiber. It can move horizontally, vertically, laterally, and rotate. Treatment couches may be indexed for increased reproducibility of treatment set-ups.

17. D. On-board imaging and other imaging used for target localization include: KV imagers with flat-panel detectors, MV imagers (electronic portal imaging devices—EPIDs) with flat-panel detectors, in room CT scanners (CT scanner on rails), KV Cone-Beam CT (KV imager is mounted to treatment machine and obtains images as it rotates around the patient), MV Cone-Beam CT (Uses EPID to capture images and images are reconstructed), helical tomotherapy, and ultrasound.

18. B. The Conventional Simulator is designed to mimic all aspects of a linear accelerator—including mechanical, geometrical and optical actions. The X-ray tube is in the gantry head of the linear accelerator.

19. C. The collimator assembly can also rotate 360° and includes blades/shutters, also known as beam-restricting diaphragms, which limit the X-ray field to improve image quality, field-defining wires which imitate field size on treatment machine, fiducial plate, which serves as method of measurement of field size and patient anatomy on image, optical distance indicator, and accessory holder.

20. B. The gantry of the CT scanner contains X-ray tubes and detectors, also referred to as the bore. The X-ray tube rotates around patient continuously as table moves. Detectors, fan beam, or fixed around the gantry are opposite of the X-ray tubes and converts radiation to light, which is then converted to an electrical signal, which is further transformed into an image.

21. B. The density of a structure is represented by CT number or Hounsfield units. Hounsfield units range from +1000 (bright white) to −1000 (dark black). Dense bone has a value of +1000, water has a value of 0, and air has a value of +1000.
22. A.
23. C. Voxels represent the slice thickness of a CT image. Window level controls the brightness of the image, while window width controls the contrast of the image.
24. B. Tomotherapy delivers radiation in a helical fashion, while components of treatment machine and/or treatment couch are moving. Cyberknife, frameless stereotactic radiosurgery equipment, is a LINAC mounted on robotic arm. This equipment treats patient precisely while continuously acquiring patient images and will only treat the patient when target is in correct location. Gamma Knife is used for stereotactic radiosurgery to the brain. This device sas 201 Cobalt−60 sources, which are collimated in order to provide high dose to target with minimal dose to normal tissue. Proton beam therapy utilized cyclotrons or synchrotrons to create proton beam, utilizing the proton's Bragg peak to dump dose at the target, without much dose to normal tissue (specifically past the target).

Suggested Readings

Armstrong J, Washington CM. Photon dosimetry concepts and calculations. In: Washington CM, Leaver D, editors. Principles and practice of radiation therapy. 3rd ed. St. Louis, MO: Mosby Elsevier; 2010. p. 492–526.

Karzmark CJ, Morton RJ. A primer on theory and operation of linear accelerators in radiation therapy. Madison, WI: Medical Physics Publishing; 1998.

Khan FM. The physics of radiation therapy. 4th ed. Baltimore, MD: Lippincott Williams & Wilkins; 2010.

Leaver D. Treatment delivery equipment. In: Washington CM, Leaver D, editors. Principles and practice of radiation therapy. 3rd ed. St. Louis, MO: Mosby Elsevier; 2010. p. 133–57.

Leaver D, Uricchio N, Griggs P. Simulator design. In: Washington CM, Leaver D, editors. Principles and practice of radiation therapy. 3rd ed. St. Louis, MO: Mosby Elsevier; 2010. p. 416–41.

Uricchio N. Computed tomography simulation. In: Washington CM, Leaver D, editors. Principles and practice of radiation therapy. 3rd ed. St. Louis, MO: Mosby Elsevier; 2010. p. 467–91.

Chapter 5
Quality Assurance

Questions

1. Ionization chambers used for the quality assurance of treatment machines should be calibrated at an Accredited Dosimetry Calibration Lab (ADCL) every _____.

    A. 6 months
    B. 1 year
    C. 2 years
    D. 5 years

2. The radiation therapy treatment chart should be checked, at minimum, on a _____ basis.

    A. Daily
    B. Weekly
    C. Monthly
    D. Annual

3. Which organization provides guidelines for facilities to follow in regards to Linear Accelerator Quality Assurance?

    A. American Society of Radiologic Technologists
    B. American Society of Radiation Oncologists
    C. American Registry of Radiologic Technologists
    D. American Association of Physicists in Medicine

4. Why are some linear accelerator quality assurance tests completed less often than others?

    A. They are unlikely to change over time
    B. Impact of malfunction is low
    C. A and B
    D. All tests are performed on a monthly basis

5. A _____ test is used to check multiple beam alignment.

    A. Split beam
    B. Collimator digital readout
    C. Cross-hair centering
    D. Gantry

6. On the linear accelerator, the door interlock should be tested:

    A. Daily
    B. Weekly
    C. Monthly
    D. Annually

7. Daily photon output constancy on the linear accelerator should be within ____% of normal limits.

    A. 1
    B. 2
    C. 3
    D. 4

8. The optical distance indicator can be measured using this tool:

    A. Localizing lasers
    B. Lutz device
    C. Mechanical distance front pointer
    D. Laser cube

9. Which of the following is the correct formula to correct for temperature and pressure changes, which would affect ionization readings?

    A. $Correction_{t,p}$ Factor $= (760/P) \times [(273+T)/295]$
    B. $Correction_{t,p}$ Factor $= (760/P)/[(273+T)/295]$
    C. $Correction_{t,p}$ Factor $= (P/760) \times [295/(273+T)]$
    D. $Correction_{t,p}$ Factor $= (P/760)/[295/(273+T)]$

10. Beam flatness is measured over ____ of field width, specified at 10 cm depth.

    A. 50 %
    B. 60 %
    C. 70 %
    D. 80 %

11. What test is completed by measuring and comparing multiple points of a beam profile equidistance from the central axis?

    A. Beam flatness
    B. Beam symmetry
    C. Radiation/light field coincidence
    D. Output constancy

12. What is the tolerance for the monthly light field/radiation field coincidence test? (Choose all correct answers).

    A. 1 mm
    B. 2 mm
    C. 1 %
    D. 2 %

13. Gantry and collimator angle indicators are checked:

    A. Daily
    B. Weekly
    C. Monthly
    D. Annual

14. Tolerance of the cross-hair centering is:

    A. 1 mm
    B. 1 %
    C. 2 mm
    D. 2 %

15. Collimator, gantry, and couch rotation around the isocenter are tested on a _____ basis.

    A. Daily
    B. Weekly
    C. Monthly
    D. Annual

16. After completing the collimator rotation around the isocenter test, the resulting exposure on the film will have the appearance of a:

    A. Star
    B. Prism
    C. Straight line
    D. Two intersecting lines

17. Which of the following is not a multileaf collimator test?

    A. Leaf shape
    B. Leaf travel
    C. Leaf speed
    D. Transmission between leaves

18. The door interlock test for the CT simulator is completed:

    A. Daily
    B. Monthly
    C. Annual
    D. There is not door interlock for CT simulators

19. Daily image quality tests for the CT simulator include verifying CT units for:

    A. Water
    B. Fat
    C. Bone
    D. All of the above

20. Table indexing on the CT simulator is checked:

    A. Daily
    B. Weekly
    C. Monthly
    D. Annually

21. When treating patients with intensity-modulated radiation therapy (IMRT), the plan must be delivered to a phantom to evaluate dose distribution prior to the:

    A. First treatment
    B. Fifth treatment
    C. Half-way mark
    D. Final treatment

22. Localizing lasers should be tested _____ and within _____ of standard.

    A. Daily, 2 %
    B. Daily, 2 mm
    C. Weekly, 2 %
    D. Weekly, 2 mm

23. In order for quality care, patients should receive at minimum of _____ of their intended dose.

    A. 1 %
    B. 2 %
    C. 5 %
    D. 10 %

24. Which of the following quality assurance tests should be completed daily on a linear accelerator? (Choose all correct answers).

    A. Beam symmetry
    B. X-ray beam output constancy
    C. Table-top sag
    D. Door interlock

25. Output constancy at different gantry angles is measured:

    A. Daily
    B. Monthly
    C. Every 6 months
    D. Annually

26. Which of the following is not a source for light field/radiation field incongruence?

    A. Misalignment of target
    B. Misalignment of table top due to sag
    C. Misalignment of mirror
    D. Misalignment of light source

27. Daily quality assurance of CT number of water for image quality of CT simulators should be within:

    A. 1 Hounsfield unit
    B. 5 Hounsfield units
    C. 10 Hounsfield units
    D. 15 Hounsfield units

28. Electron beam flatness should be within:

    A. 2 %
    B. 3 %
    C. 5 %
    D. 8 %

29. Daily output constancy for X-rays should be measured with a field size of:

    A. 5×5 cm
    B. 10×10 cm
    C. 15×15 cm
    D. 20×20 cm

Answers and Rationales

1. C. All equipment used in dose measurement must be calibrated following NRC and state licensing agreements. Ionization chambers must be calibrated every 2 years at an Accredited Dosimetry Calibration Lab (ADCL).
2. B. Radiation therapy treatment charts should be checked weekly, at minimum, as well as before third initial fraction and at completion of treatment. It should be checked for charting errors, to ensure legibility and to confirm accurate documentation.
3. D. Many facilities follow guidelines set by the American Association of Physicists in Medicine (AAPM). Task Group 40 Report was published in 1994 to provide recommendations, and have since been updated by Task Group 142 Report. CT Scanner quality assurance guidelines are also set by the AAPM.
4. C. Tests are divided into daily, monthly, and annual categories. They are also organized by dosimetry, mechanical, and safety test categories. Placement is determined by impact on the patient treatment or safety concerns in the event of a malfunction. Equipment must also be tested when a facility gets a new machine, and following repair or maintenance. Treatments should not be initiated unless all applicable tests are completed and are within tolerance limits.
5. A. Split beam test can show beam misalignment, due to focal spot displacement, asymmetry of collimator jaws, or collimator and/or gantry displacement during rotation. To perform the test, double expose a film with gantry angles 180° apart, blocking one half of the film during first exposure and the second half at second exposure. There should be no shift between two exposures.
6. A. Door interlocks are tested daily and are pass or fail. To complete, open door when beam is on or try to initiate treatment while door is open.
7. C. Tolerance for daily output constancy for electrons and photons is 3 % and is measured with output constancy tool. A 10×10 cm field is used for photons and a 10 cm cone is used for measuring output constancy for electrons.
8. C. The Optical distance indicator can be measured with a mechanical distance front pointer, or measuring from a reference point within the machine. This daily quality assurance test is very important, because if the optical distance readout is incorrect, the dose the patient receives will be altered in relationship to the inverse square law. The tolerance for the test is 2 mm.
9. A. Monthly output constancy tests are measured with an ionization chamber in solid water or a water phantom. An ionization chamber should be placed at depth within the phantom to measure output. Number of air molecules in chamber vary in density with changes in temperature and pressure. Pressure is measured in mmHg, while temperature is measured in Celsius.
10. D. Beam flatness measures field flatness over 80 % of field width, and is specified at 10 cm depth. To calculate, measure maximum and minimum dose points over a beam profile. The difference between the two points divided by their

sums is used to calculate flatness. Beam flatness can be affected by misalignment of the flattening filter.

11. B. Beam symmetry can be affected by misalignment of the flattening filter. The tolerance for both photons and electrons is 3 %.

12. B and C. Light field/radiation field coincidence is measured by using film which is packaged in a paper envelope, and taping it to treatment couch at isocenter depth. Next, mark 10×10 cm field on paper envelope and expose 10×10 cm field on film. Visually inspect radiation and light field edges to check for misalignment. The beam can be misaligned due to misalignment of target, light source or mirror.

13. C. Using a level, rotate gantry or collimator until the level indicates that the machine is in a level position—check digital angle indicator of machine. Tolerance of the test is $1°$.

14. C. To measure cross-hair centering, use a piece of paper and mark position of the cross-hair. Rotate the collimator and continue to mark the position of the cross-hair. When complete, inspect the marks and ensure that they are within tolerance. This test is completed monthly.

15. D. Collimator, gantry, and couch rotation around isocenter is measured annually. To complete the test, use film which is packaged in a paper envelope, and tape to treatment couch at isocenter depth. Open the length of the field and close the width (and vice versa), and then expose the film. Next, expose film, rotate collimator (couch or gantry) and repeat.

16. A. The film will have a starburst appearance.

17. A. Other multileaf collimator tests include projected leaf width at isocenter, leakage, and patient-specific beam shaping.

18. D. There is no door interlock for CT simulators, as interruption of the beam would require additional scans and dose to the patient (Mutic et al 2003).

19. A. In addition to checking lasers, image quality is checked daily. This test verifies CT units for water [must be within 5 Hounsfield units (HU)]. Also, image noise and spatial integrity are checked and should match manufacturer specifications (Mutic et al 2003).

20. D. Image orientation is also checked on an annual basis (Mutic et al 2003).

21. A. In addition to individual plan quality assurance, additional quality assurance should be completed on the IMRT beam delivery and treatment planning processes. Further radiation safety surveys should be completed when first implementing an IMRT program, due to the increase in monitor units used.

22. D. Selected monthly linear accelerator quality assurance procedures and tolerances are outlined in Table 5.1. Selected annual linear accelerator quality assurance procedures and tolerances are outlined in Table 5.2.

23. B. Selected monthly linear accelerator quality assurance procedures and tolerances are outlined in Table 5.1. Selected annual linear accelerator quality assurance procedures and tolerances are outlined in Table 5.2.

Table 5.1 Monthly quality assurance tolerances of linear accelerators

Test	Tolerance
X-ray output constancy	2 %
Electron output constancy	2 %
X-ray beam flatness constancy	2 %
Electron beam flatness constancy	3 %
Beam symmetry, X-ray, and electron	3 %
Light field vs. radiation field coincidence	2 mm or 1 % per side
Gantry/collimator angle indicators	1°
Cross-hair centering	2 mm
Field size indicators	2 mm
Couch position indicators	2 mm or 1°
Emergency off buttons	Functional

Source: Hendee et al. (2005), Khan (2010), Klein et al. (2009), Kutcher et al. (1994), Schneider (2010)

Table 5.2 Annual quality assurance tolerances of linear accelerators

Test	Tolerance
X-ray output constancy	2 %
Electron output constancy	2 %
Output constancy with different gantry angles, field sizes, electron applicators	2 %
Gantry, collimator, and table rotation around isocenter	2 mm
Table-top sag	2 mm

Source: Hendee et al. (2005), Khan (2010), Klein et al. (2009), Kutcher et al. (1994), Schneider (2010)

References

Hendee WR, Ibbott GS, Hendee EG. Radiation therapy physics. 3rd ed. Hoboken, NJ: Wiley; 2005.

Khan FM. The physics of radiation therapy. 4th ed. Baltimore, MD: Lippincott Williams & Wilkins; 2010.

Klein EE, Hanley J, Bayouth J, Yin FF, Simon W, Dresser S, et al. Task group 142. Med Phys. 2009;36(9):4197–212.

Kutcher GJ, Coia L, Gillin M, Hanson WF, Leibel S, Morton RJ, et al. Comprehensive QA for radiation oncology: report of AAPM Radiation Therapy Committee Task Group 40. Med Phys. 1994;21(4):581–618.

Mutic S, Palta JR, Butker EK, Das IJ, Huq MS, Loo LN, et al. Quality assurance for computed-tomography simulators and the computed-tomography-simulation process: report of the AAPM Radiation Therapy Committee Task Group No. 66. Med Phys. 2003;30(10):2762–92.

Schneider JM. Quality improvement in radiation oncology. In: Washington CM, Leaver D, editors. Principles and practice of radiation therapy. 3rd ed. St. Louis, MO: Mosby Elsevier; 2010. p. 363–75.

Chapter 6
Simulation and Treatment Planning

Questions

1. Which of the following is a negative contrast agent?

   A. Air
   B. Iodine
   C. Barium sulfate
   D. Nonionic venous contrast

2. Which of the following is not true regarding iodine contrast?

   A. Can be administered intravenously
   B. Kidney function must be checked prior to administration
   C. Is ionic only
   D. Patients allergic to shellfish should not receive iodine contrast

3. Prior to the administration of intravenous contrast, you should assess the patient for:

   A. Shellfish allergy
   B. Lung function
   C. Joint pain
   D. GI complications

4. The hyoid bone is located at what vertebral level?

   A. C1
   B. C3
   C. T1
   D. T3

© Springer Science+Business Media New York 2016
A. Heath, *Radiation Therapy Study Guide*, DOI 10.1007/978-1-4939-3258-0_6

5. The SSN corresponds to vertebral level:

   A. C3
   B. T3
   C. T6
   D. L3

6. An example of a positioning device is:

   A. Thermoplastic mask
   B. Chemical mold
   C. Head holder
   D. Vacuum mold

7. What positioning device is used to move a patient's small bowel out of pelvic treatment fields?

   A. Shoulder assistance straps
   B. Bellyboard
   C. Wingboard
   D. Thermoplastic device

8. Thermoplastic immobilization devices are used to immobilize the:

   A. Head and neck
   B. Chest
   C. Abdomen
   D. Pelvis

9. When obtaining images through conventional simulation, what is true regarding mA?

   A. Controls contrast of the image
   B. Represents the quality of the beam
   C. Controls density of the image
   D. All of the above are true

10. What is not a step of CT simulation?

    A. Scanning the area of interest per physician order
    B. Imaging with slices of 2–8 mm
    C. Taking orthogonal images
    D. Ensuring the patient anatomy and simulation marks are included in field of view as the image is reconstructed.

11. After CT simulation, what must be documented by the radiation therapist?

    A. Gantry angle
    B. Collimator angle
    C. Field size
    D. Patient setup

12. What is not included in the CTV?

    A. GTV
    B. Margin for motion
    C. Microscopic disease
    D. All of the above are included in the CTV

13. What volume accounts for the patient's physiologic movement, such as breathing?

    A. Clinical target volume
    B. Internal margin
    C. Gross target volume
    D. Motion volume

14. What term describes critical structures in or near the treatment field?

    A. Internal target volume
    B. Organs at risk
    C. Irradiated volume
    D. Internal margin

15. Which of the following is true regarding the forward planning technique?

    A. Plan is optimized after fields are designed
    B. Computer design treatment fields based on set criteria
    C. Is used for IMRT planning
    D. Is only used for brachytherapy planning.

16. Which of the following are considered when designing fields and beam arrangements? (Choose all correct answers).

    A. Total dose
    B. Beam energy
    C. Patient setup

17. Which of the following tumors would best be treated with an arc treatment?

    A. Central lung tumor
    B. Inflammatory breast cancer
    C. Ewings sarcoma
    D. Nasopharyngeal tumor

18. Which of the following beam modifying devices would not be used to compensate for missing tissue in a patient?

    A. Cerrobend blocks
    B. Bolus
    C. Compensating filters
    D. Wedges

19. Blocks are _____ HVL thick.

    A. 1
    B. 3
    C. 5
    D. 7

20. Multileaf collimators (MLC) are made of:

    A. Lipowitz metal
    B. Tungsten
    C. Lead
    D. Brass

21. What device would be used in order to compensate for missing tissue as well as increase the dose to the skin?

    A. Compensating filter
    B. Bolus
    C. Wedge
    D. Hand block

22. What is a limitation of using wedges in a patient's treatment plan?

    A. Increased time needed for treatment planning
    B. Field size limitations
    C. Limitations in gantry angles that can be used
    D. Little variety in available wedge angles

23. Calculate the hinge angle when using 30° wedges in a wedge pair field arrangement.

    A. 60°
    B. 120°
    C. 180°
    D. 240°

24. The _____ is the projection of what the treatment field will look like, from the point of view from the origin of the beam.

    A. Beam's eye view
    B. Isodose distribution
    C. Dose volume histogram
    D. Field size view

25. What is not included in the radiation therapy treatment prescription?

    A. Dose per fraction
    B. Beam-modifying devices
    C. Treatment volume
    D. Patient position

26. Calculate the equivalent square for a 6×12 cm field size.

    A. 4×4 cm
    B. 6×6 cm
    C. 8×8 cm
    D. 10×10 cm

27. The _____ factor is the ratio of dose at dmax for field size to dose at dmax for standard field size.

    A. Attenuation
    B. Output
    C. Back scatter
    D. Tissue maximum

28. Backscatter factor is the:

    A. Ratio of dose with modifier in beam to dose without modifier in beam
    B. Ratio of dose at dmax in phantom to dose at dmax in air
    C. Target-to-axis distance
    D. Ratio of absorbed dose at depth to dose at dmax

29. Percent depth dose increases with:

    A. Increased energy
    B. Decreased field size
    C. Increased depth
    D. All of the above

30. What is the Mayneord's factor for a patient who was originally treated at 100 cm SSD to a depth of 5 cm with a 10× photon beam, but now needs to be treated at 110 cm SSD?

    A. 0.990
    B. 0.993
    C. 1.003
    D. 1.010

31. The ratio of scattered dose at depth in phantom to scatter dose at depth in air is:

    A. Tissue-air ratio (TAR)
    B. Scatter-air ratio (SAR)
    C. Tissue maximum ratio (TMR)
    D. Tissue phantom ratio (TPR)

32. TAR is independent of:

    A. Energy
    B. Field size
    C. Depth
    D. SSD

33. Calculate the gap required for adjacent fields (Field A—length 12, Field B—length 20) treated at 100 cm SSD with 6 MV photon beams to a treatment depth of 5 cm.

    A. 0.5 cm
    B. 0.8 cm
    C. 1.3 cm
    D. 1.5 cm

34. Calculate the monitor units needed for a patient being treated AP/PA to their abdomen with a 12×16 cm field, SSD = 100 cm, treated midplane to a depth of 7 cm, Sc = 1.08, Sp = 1.007, %dd = 76 %, tumor dose to target is 180 cGy

    A. 90 MU
    B. 101 MU
    C. 109 MU
    D. 118 MU

35. A patient is being treated isocentrically with four fields (equally weighted) to their pelvis using 10× photons. The AP SSD is 90 cm, Right Lateral SSD is 78 cm, PA SSD is 90 cm and left lateral SSD is 82 cm. The total tumor dose per fraction is 180 cGy. What information will you need before you can look up the factors to complete the monitor unit calculation?

    A. Field size
    B. Patient position
    C. Location of patient tattoos
    D. Gantry angles

36. The practical range of a 12 MeV electron beam is:

    A. 3 cm
    B. 4 cm
    C. 6 cm
    D. 12 cm

37. How many monitor units are needed for a lumpectomy boost electron treatment, prescribed to the 80 % isodose line? The Cfs for the treatment field using a 10×10 cm cone with minimal blocking is 1.05. The dose per field is 200 cGy.

    A. 211 MU's
    B. 238 MU's
    C. 190 MU's
    D. 214 MUs

Answers and Rationales

1. A. Negative contrast shows up dark on images, as it absorbs less radiation than tissue. Oxygen and air are most common types. Positive contrast shows up light or white on images, as it absorbs more radiation than tissue. Compounds with high atomic numbers are positive contrast agents. Barium sulfate and iodine are the common types of positive contrast agents.
2. C. Iodine contrast can be ionic (increased risk for allergic reactions) or non-ionic. It is administered intravenously to visualize vessels and kidneys or through catheter into bladder.
3. A. Prior to administration, it is important to check kidney function prior, as well as questioning the patient for allergies to prior contrast and shellfish.
4. B. See Table 6.1 for commonly used external landmarks.
5. B. See Table 6.1 for commonly used external landmarks.
6. C. Positioning devices are used to help patient keep position each day and can be used for multiple patients. Examples are head holders, knee sponges, shoulder assistance straps, and wing boards. Bellyboards are used to move the patient's small bowel out of pelvic treatment fields.
7. B. See Question 6 for more details about positioning devices.
8. A. Immobilization devices are used to immobilization the patient's anatomy being treated. Historically, tape was used. Thermoplastic immobilization devices are used for immobilization of the head and neck areas. Chemical molds may be used for immobilizing chest, abdomen or pelvis, as are vacuum molds. With IMRT treatment, abdominal compression devices are used when treating chest and abdomen to immobilize tumors in this area.
9. C. Milliamperage (mA) is the quantity of beam and controls overall density. Kilovoltage potential (KvP) is the quality of beam and controls contrast. When

Table 6.1 Frequently used external landmarks

Structure	Associated vertebral body
External auditory meatus	C1
Hyoid bone	C3–C4
Thyroid cartilage	C4
Cricoid cartilage	C6
Vertebral prominance	C7
Suprasternal notch (SSN)	T2–T3
Carina	T4–T5
Xiphoid	T10
Umbilicus	L4
Bifurcation of abdominal aorta	L4
Superior iliac crest	L4

Source: Washington CM. Surface and sectional anatomy. In: Washington CM, Leaver D, editors. Principles and practice of radiation therapy. 3rd ed. St. Louis, MO: Mosby Elsevier; 2010, pp. 376–415

taking images, follow the 15 % rule—an increase of 15 % of KvP should also include a decrease of mAs by 50 %.

10. C. Orthogonal images are reconstructed after the CT simulation is completed.
11. D. Following the CT simulation procedure, the radiation therapist should document information to reproduce patient setup (position, tattoo location, positioning aids, and immobilization devices used), patient measurements, and special instructions.
12. B. After acquiring images, tumor, target, and organs at risk are identified by radiation oncologist and planning dosimetrist and/or physicist. Volumes used in treatment planning are:

- Gross tumor volume (GTV): tumor itself
- Clinical target volume (CTV): GTV + margin to include anatomy which may have microscopic disease
- Planning target volume (PTV): CTV + margin for setup uncertainty or patient movement

    - Internal margin (IM): margin to account for patient's physiologic movement
    - Internal target volume (ITV): CTV + IM

- Treated volume: anatomy receiving prescription dose
- Irradiated volume: area that receives dose significant to normal tissue tolerance
- Organs at risk (OAR): critical structures in or near treatment field

13. B. Please see question 12 for details about treatment planning volumes.
14. B. Please see question 12 for details about treatment planning volumes.
15. A. Treatment planning can be forward or inverse. With forward planning, the beams are designed and then changed to optimize the plan. With inverse planning, the computer program designs beams, based on criteria set at beginning of planning session; used for IMRT treatment planning.
16. A, B, and C. When designing fields and beam arrangements, one must consider dose and fractionation scheme, isocentric or isometric setup, modality (photons or electrons), beam energy, number of fields needed to decrease dose to normal tissue, fixed or rotational beams, field weighting, and beam attenuation in tissue. Bone attenuates radiation beam more than tissue, while lungs attenuate less.
17. A. Rotational fields are useful for central, well-defined tumors. The isocenter is set past tumor (past-pointing) to ensure point of highest dose is in the target.
18. A. Compensating filters compensate for missing tissue. The filter is made of tissue-equivalent material to a thickness equal to that of tissue missing. Compensating filters allow for improved dose distribution while preserving skin-sparing effect. Bolus is tissue equivalent material placed directly on patient skin which can be used to compensate for missing tissue or increase dose to skin. Bolus must be flat on skin and air gaps must be eliminated. Commercially

available products are most commonly used, as well as wet gauze, rice bags, and others. Wedges may also be added to compensate for missing tissue.

19. C. Blocks must transmit less than 5 % of the treatment beam, thus are 5 HVL thick. Hand blocks are non-divergent standardized blocks, which are placed in slotted block tray and placed clinically. They are useful for emergency treatments. Custom blocks are made of cerrobend, or Lipowitz metal, and are custom to patient and field. These divergent blocks can be positive (block center of field) or negative (block outside of field).

20. B. Multileaf collimators are computer controlled blocking in the treatment machine used to customize treatment fields. Made of tungsten, these devices can move during treatment to modulate treatment beam.

21. B. See Question 18 for details about compensators and bolus.

22. B. Wedges are used to alter isodose distribution in patient or compensate for sloping surfaces. Physical wedges come in 15°, 30°, 45°, and 60° angles and have field size limitations. The heel of wedge is the thicker part of wedge, while the toe is the thinner portion. When compensating for a sloping surface, the heel is placed towards area missing tissue. Dynamic wedges are when the jaw of collimator moves during treatment to simulate a wedge in treatment field.

23. B. Wedge pairs are when two fields use wedges to modify the isodose distribution. The hinge angle is angle between two fields. The formula for hinge angle $= 180° - (2 \times$ wedge angle). When using wedge pairs, heels are placed together.

24. A. Fields and beam arrangements are evaluated with several tools. The beam's eye view (BEV) is the projection of what the treatment field will look like, from point of view from the origin of beam. Isodose distributions are graphical representation of how dose is deposited within the tissue. Dose volume histograms (DVH) are graphical representation of volume of organ vs. dose received.

25. D. The radiation therapy treatment prescription must include treatment volume and dose, fractionation scheme (number of fractions, dose per fraction and scheduling of fractions), information regarding treatment (mode and energy of radiation and beam modifying devices).

26. C. The equivalent square of treatment fields is used for dose calculations. This takes into account different scattering properties of different shaped fields. Equivalent square of field $= 4 \times$ (area of field/perimeter of field).

27. B. Output factor is the ratio of dose at dmax for field size to dose at dmax for standard field size (typically 10×10 cm). Output factor may also be referred to as Sc (collimator scatter factor) and is typically 1 cGy/MU at dmax with 10×10 cm field. Output factor increases with increased field size.

28. B. Backscatter factor (BSF) is the ratio of dose at dmax in phantom to dose at dmax in air, and may be referred to as peak scatter factor. BSF is dependent of energy and field size but independent of SSD. Sp (phantom scatter factor) = ratio of BSF for given field to BSF for reference field (usually 10×10 cm). Attenuation factor is the ratio of dose with modifier in beam to dose without modifier in beam and used for wedges, block trays, and compensators. Percent depth dose is the ratio of absorbed dose at depth to dose at dmax.

29. A. Percent depth dose increases with increased energy, increases with increased field size, decreases with increased depth, and decreases with increased SSD.

30. C. Mayneord's factor is used for SSD calculation when the patient is treated with a different SSD:

$$MF = \left\{ (SSD_1 + d)/(SSD_1 + d\max) \right\}^2 \times \left\{ (SSD_2 + d\max)/(SSD_2 + d) \right\}^2$$

31. B. Tissue-air ratio (TAR) is the ratio of dose at depth in phantom to dose at depth in air. Scatter-air ratio (SAR) is the ratio of scattered dose at depth in phantom to scatter dose at depth in air and used for irregularly shaped fields. Tissue maximum ratio (TMR) is the ratio of dose at depth to dose at dmax, while tissue-phantom ratio (TPR) is the ratio of dose at depth to dose at reference depth.

32. D. TAR increases with increased energy and increased field size, decreases with increased depth, and is independent of SSD. This factor is used in SAD calculations. TAR=BSF when measured at dmax.

33. B. To calculate the skin gap of adjacent photon fields, use the following formula:

$$\text{Gap} = \left[(L_{1/2}) \times (d/SSD_1) \right] + \left[(L_{2/2}) \times (d/SSD_2) \right]$$

34. C. To calculate monitor units for SSD treatments, use the following formula:

$$MU = \frac{\text{Tumor dose per treatment field}}{1cGy/MU \times Sc \times Sp \times \%dd \times SSD\,factor \times attenuation\,factors}$$

$$SSD\,factor = \left[SCD/(SSD + d\max) \right]^2$$

35. A. To calculate monitor units for SAD treatments, use the following formula:

$$MU = \frac{\text{Tumor dose per treatment field}}{1cGy/MU \times Sc \times Sp \times TMR \times SAD\,factor \times attenuation\,factors}$$

$$SAD\,factor = (SCD/SAD)^2$$

36. C. Range of electrons is based on energy. The practical range (Rp) is the depth electrons travel in tissue, and is calculated by MeV of beam/2. The depth of 80 % isodose curve=MeV of beam/3, while the depth of 90 % isodose curve=MeV of beam/4.

37. B. Information used in electron calculations include tumor dose per fraction, depth of target, cone size and blocking factors (Cfs), and calibration factor (Ccal) (typically 1 cGy/MU).

To calculate monitor units for electron treatments, use the following formula:

$$MU = \frac{\text{Tumor dose per treatment field}}{\text{Prescription}\,\%dd \times Cfs \times Ccal}$$

Suggested Readings

Armstrong J, Washington CM. Photon dosimetry concepts and calculations. In: Washington CM, Leaver D, editors. Principles and practice of radiation therapy. 3rd ed. St. Louis, MO: Mosby Elsevier; 2010. p. 492–526.

Bass LH, Anderson SL. Infection control in radiation oncology facilities. In: Washington CM, Leaver D, editors. Principles and practice of radiation therapy. 3rd ed. St. Louis, MO: Mosby Elsevier; 2010. p. 190–225.

Hendee WR, Ibbott GS, Hendee EG. Radiation therapy physics. 3rd ed. Hoboken, NJ: Wiley; 2005.

Kempa AF. Electron beams in radiation therapy. In: Washington CM, Leaver D, editors. Principles and practice of radiation therapy. 3rd ed. St. Louis, MO: Mosby Elsevier; 2010. p. 550–63.

Khan FM. The physics of radiation therapy. 4th ed. Baltimore, MD: Lippincott Williams & Wilkins; 2010.

Leaver D, Keller R, Uricchia N. Conventional (fluoroscopy-based) simulation procedures. In: Washington CM, Leaver D, editors. Principles and practice of radiation therapy. 3rd ed. St. Louis, MO: Mosby Elsevier; 2010. p. 442–66.

Stanton R, Stinson D. Applied physics for radiation oncology. Madison, WI: Medical Physics Publishing; 1996.

Urrichio N. Computed tomography simulation. In: Washington CM, Leaver D, editors. Principles and practice of radiation therapy. 3rd ed. St. Louis, MO: Mosby Elsevier; 2010. p. 467–91.

Vassil AD, Videtic GMM. Tools for simulation and treatment. In: Videtic GMM, Vassil AD, editors. Handbook of treatment planning in radiation oncology. New York: Demos Medical Publishing; 2011. p. 15–24.

Washington CM. Surface and sectional anatomy. In: Washington CM, Leaver D, editors. Principles and practice of radiation therapy. 3rd ed. St. Louis, MO: Mosby Elsevier; 2010. p. 376–415.

Wuu CS. Three-dimensional physics and treatment planning. In: Chao KSC, Perez CA, Brady LW, editors. Radiation oncology management decisions. 3rd ed. Philadelphia, PA: Wolters Kluwer-Lippincott Williams and Wilkins; 2011. p. 31–40.

Chapter 7
Treatment Delivery

Questions

1. Which is not true regarding patient positioning?

    A. Patient comfort is not important if the patient is immobilized
    B. Patients may need to remove dentures or other devices prior to treatment
    C. Documentation of patient setup is necessary for daily positioning
    D. Positioning must be verified daily

2. When three-pointing a patient, the patient is positioned in all of the following planes except:

    A. W
    B. X
    C. Y
    D. Z

3. Orthogonal films are two films taken _____ degrees apart.

    A. 45
    B. 90
    C. 180
    D. 275

4. Which modality of radiation therapy measures movement of the tumor?

    A. 2D
    B. 3D
    C. 4D
    D. IMRT

© Springer Science+Business Media New York 2016
A. Heath, *Radiation Therapy Study Guide*, DOI 10.1007/978-1-4939-3258-0_7

5. Dose calculations must have _____ independent checks prior to initial treatment.

    A. One
    B. Two
    C. Three
    D. Four

6. Which of the following checks is necessary for arc radiation therapy treatment but not static radiation therapy treatment?

    A. Couch indexing
    B. Patient positioning
    C. Use of correct patient marks
    D. Clearance of gantry and table

7. Which of the following is not necessary to be included in a radiation therapy prescription?

    A. Anatomic site
    B. Treatment technique
    C. Side effect management teaching
    D. Fractionation schedule

8. Which of the following treatment machine components must the radiation therapists check prior to treatment? (Choose all correct answers).

    A. Optical distance indicator
    B. Machine parameters
    C. Field light operation
    D. Patient positioning

9. Which of the following are indications for patient monitoring during treatment? (Choose all correct answers).

    A. Patient safety
    B. Watch for patient motion
    C. Prevent collision of gantry and table

10. Patient monitoring should include (Choose all correct answers):

    A. Two-way audio communication
    B. Visual contact with patient's treatment area
    C. MLC movement for IMRT
    D. Visual contact with patient monitors in the event of anesthesia

11. What is not a parameter verified by all record and verify software systems?

    A. Beam positioning (gantry, collimator, table)
    B. Correct patient
    C. Field size and/or cone size
    D. Monitor units

12. At minimum, verification imaging should be completed (Choose all that apply):

    A. At the beginning of the course of treatment
    B. Every fraction
    C. When changes are made to patient positioning or the treatment plan

13. Which of the following is not true regarding patient dose verification?

    A. May be completed through the use of TLDs
    B. Must be ordered by physicians
    C. Likely to be completed towards the end of a patient's course of treatment
    D. May be completed through the use of diodes

14. In the event a treatment beam was terminated due to machine malfunction, where would you be able to find the monitor units delivered to the patient?

    A. Backup monitor unit counter
    B. From physics staff
    C. Only available through record and verify computer
    D. Electrical circuit breaker box

15. Unintended table movement during treatment is an example of:

    A. Mechanical malfunction
    B. Radiation malfunction
    C. Electrical malfunction
    D. Human error

16. If the beam fails to terminate after the appropriate amount of monitor units have been delivered, what is the first thing a radiation therapist should do?

    A. Push emergency off in the treatment room
    B. Call physics staff
    C. Push beam off on the treatment console
    D. Get the patient off the table

Answers and Rationales

1. A. Prior to treatment, the radiation therapist must verify patient position and immobilization devices. This should be verified through set-up instructions, images or diagrams of the patient setup and surface anatomy as applicable. Patients should be over the correct area of the treatment couch, and any dentures or other devices which would interfere with the treatment application should be removed. In addition, the radiation therapist must ensure that patient is immobilized, yet comfortable.
2. A. Tattoos or markings from simulation are used to identify isocenter. The isocenter is triangulated by three-pointing patient, or positioning the patient in horizontal, lateral, and vertical planes (X, Y, and Z planes).
3. B. The isocenter of the treatment fields are verified prior to treatment with imaging. For IMRT and 3D treatments, orthogonal fields are used to verify isocenter (two images taken 90° apart). Radiation therapists may need to image fiducial markers (either implanted in patient or on positioning device) to localize the target.
4. C. 2D treatments are planned from 2D imaging and verified through orthogonal films and comparing to simulation films. 3D treatments are planned from 3D imaging and verified through comparing imaging to treatment plan. The number of fields vary and often have beam modifying devices. With 4D treatments, movement (tumor, breathing) is measured and must be verified on the first day of treatment. IMRT is an advanced form of 3D CRT which shapes dose around the tumor volume while sparing OARs. The plan is verified by intensity map prior to treatment.
5. B. Dose calculations must have two independent checks prior to treatment. Radiation therapists must also review the calculation prior to treatment. In addition, the radiation therapists should check field sizes, beam modifiers, and treatment depth. Blocking and positioning of each treatment portal should be verified with the beam's eye view of each portal (typically in form of digitally reconstructed radiograph). Prescription and treatment plan must be verified prior to treatment daily to ensure no changes have been made.
6. D. If treating with arc therapy, must verify gantry and imagers clear patient and all equipment within the room.
7. C. While side effect management teaching is a required portion of the patient chart, it is not required in the treatment prescription.
8. A, B, and C. While patient positioning must be verified prior to treatment, it is not a machine component. Machine components that should be reviewed and verified include daily quality assurance tests, cone interlocks, collimator and gantry functions, field light, treatment couch operation, optical distance indicator, and machine control panel lights. Machine parameters must also be checked, such as gantry and collimator parameters, field size, beam modifiers, and mode and energy of the beam. Correct patient and site must be verified prior to treatment in daily time out procedure.

9. A, B, and C. Patients must be monitored at all times while in the room and during their treatment. Reasons for monitoring include patient safety (watch patient for distress, indicating an emergency situation), to avoid geometric miss of tumor caused by patient motion (voluntary or involuntary), to provide a visual double checking of setup, and to prevent collision of gantry and table when movement during or between treatments.

10. A, B, C, and D. Direct monitoring of the patient is not common in radiation oncology due to the shielding needed for megavoltage treatment. Leaded glass windows are available for patient monitoring in the simulation rooms, as well as any orthovoltage treatment rooms. Two cameras should be used to provide video contact of the patient, one focused on the area being treated and one to monitor patient in the event they are distressed. If a patient is anesthetized, additional video contact should remain on the patient's vital monitors. Two-way audio contact should also be part of patient monitoring. Radiation therapists should also monitor MLC movement for IMRT treatments.

11. B. Record and verify software systems are used in radiation oncology to verify and record treatment parameters each fraction. Information is inputted from the treatment plan and verified prior to treatment. These parameters include monitor units, beam positioning (gantry, collimator, table), use of beam modifiers, field size, and/or cone size, and type of radiation and energy. Treatment beam initiation is prevented if parameters are outside set tolerance limits.

12. A and C. Portal imaging provides record of the patient's treatment. At minimum, verification imaging should be completed at the beginning of the course of treatment, every five fractions, when changes are made to patient positioning or the treatment plan and as indicated by the physician. Images should include treatment portal, as well as surrounding anatomy (double-exposed images).

13. C. Patient dose may be verified by the use of TLDs, diodes or film the first few fractions of treatment. Physicians must provide orders for the additional monitoring of dose.

14. A. Radiation therapists should document the following after a machine malfunction: date and time of occurrence, description of problem and actions taken, and monitor units patient received (found in backup counter in treatment machine console).

15. A. In the event of a patient emergency or equipment malfunction, radiation therapists must be aware of the types of malfunction and actions to take. Radiation malfunctions include irregular or very slow dose rate or the machine fails to stop at the end of the prescribed dose. Electrical malfunctions may be power outages or interruptions, or irregularities in current may cause circuit breakers to trip. Mechanical malfunctions may be unintended movement of table, gantry or collimators.

16. C. The beam should terminate after the appropriate amount of monitor units has been delivered. If that does not occur, then the backup timer should terminate the beam. If the beam continues, one should:

- Push beam off/reset/turn key
- Push emergency off on console

- Turn off circuit breaker
- Open door
- Push emergency off in room
- Get patient off table and out of room
- Close the door
- Alert proper staff (physics, biomedical engineering) and keep others from entering the room

Suggested Readings

Coleman AM. Treatment procedures. In: Washington CM, Leaver D, editors. Principles and practice of radiation therapy. 3rd ed. St. Louis, MO: Mosby Elsevier; 2010. p. 158–79.

Galvin J, Blumberg AL, Camphausen K, Hayden SE, Kuettel M, Rivard MJ, et al. The process of care in radiation oncology. In: Zietman AL, Palta JR, Steinberg ML, editors. Safety is no accident. A framework for quality radiation oncology and care. Fairfax, VA: American Society for Radiation Oncology; 2012. p. 3–10.

Leaver D. Treatment delivery equipment. In: Washington CM, Leaver D, editors. Principles and practice of radiation therapy. 3rd ed. St. Louis, MO: Mosby Elsevier; 2010. p. 133–57.

Marks LB, Pavord D, Burns RA, Dawson LA, Kachnic LA, Johnston PAS, et al. Safety. In: Zietman AL, Palta JR, Steinberg ML, editors. Safety is no accident. A framework for quality radiation oncology and care. Fairfax, VA: American Society for Radiation Oncology; 2012. p. 19–27.

Stanton R, Stinson D. Applied physics for radiation oncology. Madison, WI: Medical Physics Publishing; 1996.

Chapter 8
Principles of Patient Care

Questions

1. The use of verbal communication between a patient and caregiver may be affected by:

    A. Patient's hearing ability
    B. Caregiver educational level
    C. Patient's ability to understand English
    D. A and B
    E. A and C
    F. A, B and C

2. The use of facial expressions, gestures, and proxemics to communicate is categorized as:

    A. Verbal communication
    B. Written communication
    C. Nonverbal communication
    D. Physical communication

3. Race describes:

    A. Learned behaviors passed on from one generation to the next in a specific society
    B. Persons having similar physical characteristics
    C. Definition of health and illness
    D. A and B
    E. B and C

© Springer Science+Business Media New York 2016
A. Heath, *Radiation Therapy Study Guide*, DOI 10.1007/978-1-4939-3258-0_8

4. Which of the following is not affected by a patient's cultural background?

A. Communication patterns
B. Access to healthcare
C. Method of treatment of different diseases
D. All of the above are affected

5. According to Elizabeth Kubler-Ross, the final stage of dealing with death/loss is

A. Bargaining
B. Denial
C. Anger
D. Acceptance

6. Which of the following behaviors are helpful when speaking with patients who are hard of hearing? (Choose all correct answers).

A. Yell at patient
B. Speak slower
C. Face patient when speaking
D. Only use written communication

7. Which group of children learns by playing?

A. Infants
B. Toddlers
C. School age
D. Adolescents

8. Decreased fear and anxiety and increased patient compliance can be achieved by:

A. Informal consent
B. Patient education
C. Joint Commission Accreditation
D. Privacy

9. When providing patient education to the patient, which of the following is not necessary?

A. Necessary preparation for procedure
B. The simulation or treatment process, including explanation of purpose of procedure and mechanics of the procedure
C. Provider's education and background
D. Length of the procedure

10. What is a normal rectal temperature?

A. 97.6 °F
B. 98.6 °F
C. 99.6 °F
D. 100.6 °F

11. If measuring a patient's respirations, which of the following would be within normal limits?

    A. 10 breaths per minute
    B. 16 breaths per minute
    C. 20 breaths per minute
    D. 26 breaths per minute

12. If measuring a patient's pulse, which of the following would be within normal limits?

    A. 50 beats per minute
    B. 80 beats per minute
    C. 50 beats per second
    D. 80 beats per second

13. Blood pressure is measured using a(n):

    A. Oximeter
    B. Barometer
    C. Sphygmomanometer
    D. Ecg lead

14. A normal value for diastolic blood pressure is:

    A. 30 mmHg
    B. 60 mmHg
    C. 90 mmHg
    D. All of the above are within normal limits

15. Acute side effects are those that last for ___ or less:

    A. 18 months
    B. 12 months
    C. 6 months
    D. 1 month

16. The severity of a patient's side effects depends on:

    A. Area treated
    B. Volume of organ treated
    C. Calendar month patient is treated in
    D. A and B
    E. A, B, C

17. Which of the following is not a general side effect?

    A. Skin reaction
    B. Fatigue
    C. Diarrhea
    D. Anorexia

18. A Stage III skin reaction would be characterized by:

    A. Dry desquamation
    B. Moist desquamation
    C. Necrosis
    D. Erythema

19. Which of the following is not an example of a chronic radiation side effect of the skin?

    A. Dry desquamation
    B. Fibrosis
    C. Lymphedema
    D. Telangiectasia

20. In order to minimize skin reactions, patients undergoing radiation therapy should avoid (Choose all correct answers):

    A. Sun and wind exposure to treatment site
    B. Moisturizers containing alcohol
    C. Mild cleansers

21. Extreme tiredness, difficulty being able to continue normal activities of daily living or work, and muscle weakness can be described as:

    A. Sepsis
    B. Anorexia
    C. Fatigue
    D. Cachexia

22. Lack of appetite is defined as:

    A. Marasmus
    B. Anorexia
    C. Kwashiorkor
    D. Fatigue

23. Temporary alopecia can be seen in doses around:

    A. 5 Gy
    B. 15 Gy
    C. 35 Gy
    D. 55 Gy

24. Treatment of pneumonitis may include the use of:

    A. Antibiotics
    B. Antiviral drugs
    C. Humidifier
    D. Antiemetic

25. Destruction of epithelial cells in the stomach results in _____, and begins at doses around_____.

    A. Diarrhea, 1000–2000 cGy
    B. Nausea, 1000–2000 cGy
    C. Diarrhea, 2000–3000 cGy
    D. Nausea, 2000–3000 cGy

26. Which of the following is not a treatment for nausea and vomiting?

    A. Eating small meals
    B. Eating bland foods
    C. Eating cold foods
    D. Eating spicy foods

27. Destruction of the intestinal villi results in:

    A. Diarrhea
    B. Vomiting
    C. Erythema
    D. All of the above

28. Which of the following is not recommended for patients following a low-residue diet?

    A. Whole-wheat products
    B. Cooked vegetables
    C. Low-fat dairy
    D. Lean protein (poultry)

29. Thrombocytopenia is a decrease in:

    A. Platelets
    B. White blood cells
    C. Red blood cells
    D. Stem cells

30. Which of the following blood values is not in normal range?

    A. RBC count: 3.2 million/mm^3
    B. WBC count: 7000/mm^3
    C. Platelets: 400,000/mm^3
    D. Hemoglobin: 14.5/100 ml

31. What term is used to describe the generalized symptom of wasting away?

    A. Marasmus
    B. Anemia
    C. Cachexia
    D. Asepsis

32. A long-term side effect of treatment to the salivary glands is:

    A. Thrush
    B. Inflammation
    C. Xerostomia
    D. Odynophagia

33. Thrush may be treated with:

    A. Antiemetics
    B. Antifungal infections
    C. Antibiotics
    D. Corticosteroids

34. Marasmus is:

    A. General state of wasting away
    B. Calorie malnutrition
    C. Protein malnutrition
    D. Anemia

35. Patients needing continuous care would have a KPS of:

    A. 25
    B. 50
    C. 75
    D. 100

36. Hospice care is indicated for patients who:

    A. Have less than 6 months life expectancy
    B. Do not require daily care
    C. Have financial problems
    D. All of the above

37. Which of the following patients would be at greatest risk for a pathologic fracture?

    A. Blastic bone metastasis
    B. Lytic bone metastasis
    C. Brain metastasis
    D. Lung metastasis

38. When aiding an ambulatory patient to the treatment table, where should you walk?

    A. In front of the patient
    B. Behind the patient
    C. On the patient's weak side
    D. On the patient's strong side

39. What device may be used to move patient who cannot stand from a wheelchair to the treatment table?

    A. Slider board
    B. Hoyer lift
    C. Transfer board
    D. Gait belt

40. When patients arrive to the radiation therapy department on a cart, what device is useful to help transfer patients to the treatment table?

    A. Slider board
    B. Gait belt
    C. Knee pillow
    D. Safety assistance straps

41. When patients arrive to the radiation therapy department with an infusion pump, the bag containing the medicine should be placed:

    A. On the patient's IV site
    B. Above the patient's IV site
    C. Below the patient's IV site
    D. Position of the bag does not matter

42. Chest tube drainage collection containers should be placed:

    A. On the patient's chest
    B. Above the patient's chest
    C. Below the patient's chest
    D. Position of the container does not matter

43. This medical intervention may be used in patients being treated with radiation to the head and neck area to ensure proper nutrition during treatment:

    A. Gastrostomy
    B. PICC Line
    C. Tracheostomy
    D. Foley catheter

44. Which of the following is not a reason for bladder catheterization?

    A. Visualize the bladder for treatment planning
    B. Deliver chemotherapy for bladder cancer
    C. Bypass urinary obstruction
    D. Indicate the location of the vulva for treatment planning

45. Which of the following is a normal reaction felt by patients after contrast administration?

    A. Feeling of warmth
    B. Headache
    C. Vertigo
    D. Nausea

46. If a patient is experiencing a mild reaction due to contrast administration, what symptoms may they have? (Choose all correct answers).

    A. Urticaria
    B. Nausea and vomiting
    C. Wheezing
    D. Chills
    E. Headache

47. This class of medication should be on hand when administering contrast, in the event that a patient experiences an allergic reaction:

    A. Corticosteroid
    B. Antihistamine
    C. Antiemetic
    D. Diuretic

48. With regard to cardiopulmonary resuscitation, what does CAB stand for?

    A. Circulation, airway, blood pressure
    B. Compression, AED, breathing
    C. Compression, airway, breathing
    D. Circulation, AED, blood pressure

49. Which is the correct technique to clear an airway obstruction of an unconscious person?

    A. Heimlich maneuver
    B. Abdominal thrusts
    C. Back slaps
    D. CPR

50. Signs and symptoms of a cerebral vascular accident (stroke) include (Choose all correct answers):

    A. Numbness or weakness of the face or extremities, especially on one side of the body
    B. Confusion, trouble speaking or understanding
    C. Hypoglycemia
    D. Difficulty seeing in one or both eyes

51. If you are with a patient experiencing a seizure, what action should you not take?

    A. Watch patient for aspiration
    B. Maintain patient's airway
    C. Sweep patient's mouth to ensure nothing is in oral cavity
    D. Protect patient from falls

52. Hyperglycemia is marked by:

    A. Gradual onset of polydipsia and polyuria
    B. Cold, pale, and clammy skin
    C. Seizures
    D. Dizziness

53. A patient with active tuberculosis would arrive to the radiation oncology department under _____ precautions.

    A. Contact
    B. Airborne
    C. Protective
    D. Droplet

54. Hospital acquired infections are referred to as _____ infections.

    A. Nosocomial
    B. Autoimmune
    C. Bacterial
    D. Drug resistant

55. The most effective method of decreasing hospital acquired infections is:

    A. Asceptic technique
    B. Standard precautions
    C. Handwashing
    D. Contact precautions

56. Personal protective equipment used for transmission based precautions include all of the following except:

    A. Goggles
    B. Gowns
    C. Gloves
    D. Hair coverings

57. Clostridium difficile (C Diff) spread via:

    A. Direct contact
    B. Droplets
    C. Particulate
    D. Airborne

Answers and Rationales

1. E. Verbal communication, or the exchange of information using words, may be affected by the patient's ability to hear, the patient's understanding of English (may need translator), the patient's educational level, and their ability to understand their diagnosis and medical terms.
2. C. Nonverbal communication includes body language, facial expressions, eye contact, gestures, proxemics, physical appearance, touch, and silence. Nonverbal communication is believed over verbal when there is conflict in a message.
3. B. Race describes persons having similar physical characteristics, while culture describes learned behaviors common to a given human society, passed from one generation to the next. Ethnicity illustrates multidimensional factors which include race, origin, language, religion.
4. D. In addition, culture affects healthcare through hygiene and self-care practices, attitude about immunization and other treatments, and disproportion of incidence of disease, treatment and outcomes. Understanding a patients' culture can lead to better care, because the radiation therapist can understand their patient's view on disease and treatment, as well as preferences for interactions. It is important that the radiation therapist be inclusive of cultures, yet not stereotype.
5. D. In order, the five stages are denial, anger, bargaining, depression, and acceptance.
6. B and C. While it is helpful to provide patients written instructions, this should be in addition to verbal communication as well. With the hard of hearing patients, speak slower, louder (without yelling) and face the patient in the event that they lip read. If deaf, provide the patient a sign language interpreter.
7. B. Toddlers learn by playing, so radiation therapists should use play to teach about procedures. Toddlers also fear abandonment, so using toys from home will help these patients feel more at ease.
8. B. There is much to be gained by the patient and the radiation therapist with good patient education. While patient education is required (legally and ethically), the benefits of patient education also include making patients feel more in control, and better treatment effectiveness, efficiency, and outcomes. Methods of patient education include one on one explanation, group instruction, discussions/support groups, demonstration (i.e., skin care), role-playing, programmed study, computerized learning packages, written materials, videos, and Internet guides.
9. C. Other information the radiation therapist should share with the patient are: positioning and immobilization aids and techniques and importance, as well as equipment that will be used; comfort issues related to what they can expect to hear, see, feel, smell; process of patient monitoring; follow-up care necessary, as well as side effects they may experience.

10. C. The normal axillary temperature is 97.6 °F, and normal oral temperature is 98.6 °F.
11. B. The normal range for respirations is 15–20 breaths per minute.
12. B. A normal pulse rate is 60–90 beats per minute.
13. C. Blood pressure is measured with sphygmomanometer.
14. B. Blood pressure is measure as systolic pressure (contraction of left ventricle) over diastolic pressure (relaxation of left ventricle). It is measured in mmHg, with the normal range is 90–120 mmHg/50–70 mmHg.
15. C. Side effects are considered to be acute if they last for 6 months or less. Late effects are those which occur 6 months or later following treatment.
16. D. Radiation will have an effect on normal tissue in the radiation field. The severity of the effect depends upon the area treated, dose, volume, and the patient's general condition.
17. C. Diarrhea is a specific side effect.
18. B. Stage 1 skin reaction, erythema (inflammation), occur at doses of 2000–4000 cGy. Stage 2 skin reaction, dry desquamation, occur at doses of 4000–6000 cGy. Stage 3 skin reaction is moist desquamation, while Stage 4 is marked by ulceration and necrosis. Cause of skin reactions by radiation may be attributed to damage to basal layer (stratum basale) of epidermis, redness caused by increased blood flow in healing effort, or damaged sebaceous glands.
19. A. Late or chronic skin effects include fibrosis, atrophy, necrosis, lymphedema, and telangiectasia.
20. A and B. Management of skin reactions is typically physician preference. However, general skin care practices which are helpful in all stages of skin reactions include gentle cleansing with mild soap, avoiding sun and wind exposure, as well as heat, cold, chlorinated water, perfumes, cosmetics, tape, and harsh fabrics, and using non-alcohol moisturizers after treatment. For Stage II and III reactions, patients should expose the skin to air as possible, and use topical steroids or other dressings for moist desquamation.
21. C. Fatigue is often experienced by radiation therapy patients. It is caused by the body's energy being used to heal radiation damage, anemia, malnutrition, and cancer itself. To manage fatigue, patients should make sure to get enough rest, pace activities, take in plenty of fluids, and get light to moderate physical activity or exercise.
22. B. Anorexia, or lack of appetite, can be caused by fatigue or increased waste in the bloodstream. Management of anorexia should include weighing patients regularly, and instructing patients to increase calorie and protein intake, eat many small meals, and get rest.
23. B. Hair loss in the area of treatment, due to destruction of the hair follicle, may begin about 2–3 weeks into treatment. In addition to alopecia, the patient's skin or scalp may be sore as well. This destruction is temporary from 15 to 30 Gy, however alopecia may become permanent with doses between 32 and 48 Gy. Management of alopecia includes gentle cleansing or hair, may get wig prior to needing it, avoiding heat and styling tools.

24. C. Symptoms and signs include cough, dyspnea, fever, and weakness. Diagnosed through X-rays, this side effect is caused by radiation destruction of lung tissue, specifically the alveoli. Management include rest, medicine, oxygen, and use of a humidifier.
25. B. Nausea and vomiting can occur at doses of 1000–2000 cGy when radiation fields include esophagus, stomach, or other portions of the upper abdomen. This side effect is caused by destruction of stomach epithelial cells, though it can also be caused by radiation or cancer effect on the true vomiting center in the brain.
26. D. Management may also include anti-emetic medication such as Compazine or Zofran. In addition, patients should avoid eating 1–2 h before or after treatment.
27. A. Diarrhea, marked by frequent, watery stools, and abdominal cramping can occur at doses of 2000–5000 cGy.
28. A. Examples of food allowed on a low residue diet include: white bread, cooked fruits and vegetables, low fat dairy, and lean protein.
29. A. Myelosuppression results in thrombocytopenia (decrease in platelets) which can lead to bleeding, anemia (decrease in red blood cells), and leukopenia (decrease in white blood cells) can lead to infections.
30. A. Normal blood values are outlined in Table 8.1.
31. C. Cachexia results in electrolyte and water imbalance, marked by loss of weight, muscle and fat, as well as tissue wasting and decreased quality of life.
32. C. Mouth changes occur between 1000 and 4000 cGy and can be permanent after 4000 cGy. Xerostomia is caused by damage to salivary glands, patients may find relief by using Salagen to stimulate saliva. Other side effects include mucositis, due to damage to epithelial tissues, fungal infections (Candida or thrush), or damage to taste buds located on tongue, soft palate, and pharynx.
33. B. Examples include Nystatin or Mycostatin.
34. B. Marasmus is the term to describe calorie malnutrition, while kwashiorkor describes a protein malnutrition.
35. B. Karnofsky Performance Status, or KPS, can be used to identify how pain or disease effects the patient's behavior. Normal behavior, needing no assistance,

Table 8.1 Normal blood values

Red blood cells	4.8–5.4 Million/mm^3
Hemoglobin	12–15 g/100 ml in females and 14–16.5 g/100 ml in males
Hematocrit	38–46 % in females and 40–54 % in males
White blood cells	5000–10,000/mm^3 1. 60–70 % neutrophils 2. 20–25 % lymphocytes 3. 3–8 % monocytes 4. 2–4 % eosinophils 5. 0.5–1 % basophils
Platelets	250,000–400,000/mm^3

is a KPS of 100. A KPS of 50 describes a patient who needs frequent medical care, while a KPS of 30 describes a patient who needs hospitalization.

36. A. Hospice care is indicated for patients who have a life expectancy of less than 6 months. The Medicare hospice benefit pays for all care managed by hospice during that time for qualified persons.

37. B. Lytic lesions are destructive to bone, and make bones susceptible to pathologic fractures.

38. C. You should walk alongside patient and be ready to help by assisting patients on their weak side. If the patient faints or falls, help to ease gently to the ground. You should not try to catch or hold up the patient.

39. B. For patients who can stand, place your feet between theirs and use a gait belt to help lift and pivot. In addition to a Hoyer lift, a fireman lift with one to three people may also be used for patients who are unable to stand.

40. A. Sliding boards are useful as long as patient rolling cannot cause injury. At least two people (preferably three to four) are needed for a transfer. If the patient cannot be rolled, they should be transferred with a sheet lift. In this case four to six lifters are needed with two at each side, one at head and foot; or three on each side.

41. B. Infusion catheters and pumps are used for IV delivery of chemo or other medication. Central lines (PICC, Groshong, Ports) are used for long term access to the venous system. The bag should remain 3 ft above the site of entry. Tubing should be free and unkinked. Radiation therapists should monitor IV site for infiltration (swelling, hardness, pain, coldness) and thrombophlebitis (redness, warmth, tenderness).

42. C. Chest tubes are used to remove air or fluid from the thoracic cavity, allowing lungs to re-inflate. Tubes must be kept intact, not clamped or kinked. Drainage collection container must be kept below the chest and must be kept upright to prevent backflow.

43. A. Gastrostomies allow nutrition to be directly provided into the stomach. Nasogastric tubes may also be used to provide nutrition.

44. D. Radiation therapists should keep the catheter and bag lower than the patient's bladder to prevent backflow, which may cause infection.

45. A. Patients may also report a metallic taste in their mouth. The reactions may be immediate or delayed, so monitoring patients is of utmost importance.

46. B, D, and E. Mild allergic reactions are marked by chills, coughing, dizziness, headache, nausea and mild vomiting. Moderate allergic reaction may cause erythema, urticaria (hives), bronchospasm, severe vomiting, hypertension or hypotension, and pulse changes. Severe allergic reactions produce dysphagia, constriction of throat, syncope, wheezing, convulsions, cardiac arrest or anaphylactic shock, and unresponsiveness.

47. B. Antihistamines are used for moderate allergic reactions. In the event of a severe allergic reaction, radiation therapists should have a crash cart with epinephrine and be prepared to administer CPR.

48. C. If a patient is not breathing or has no pulse, start CAB of CPR (compression, airway, breathing) and activate emergency system. Current American Heart

Association guidelines are 30 compressions to the chest followed by two breaths. An AED should be attached and used as soon as possible.

49. B. Heimlich maneuver can be used on conscious victims. To complete this, reach arms around the patient from their back, and place one closed fist inferior to the xyphoid process, covered with other hand. Pull hand in and up to put pressure on lungs, repeat as necessary. Abdominal thrusts should be used for unconscious victims. Position yourself by straddling the lower abdomen of person lying on his/her back. Using heel of hand inferior to xyphoid covered with other heel of hand, push posteriorly and superiorly three times. Check mouth to see if object has been dislodged and repeat as needed.

50. A, B, and D. Other signs and symptoms include difficulty walking, dizziness, loss of balance or coordination or sudden, severe headaches.

51. C. Seizures can be caused by tumor, stroke, hypoglycemia, hypoxia, drugs, or disease. Patients experience jerky muscle movements, loss of consciousness and incontinence during seizures. Management include maintenance of airway (do not put anything in patient's mouth), protection of patient from injury (i.e., falling off table), and rolling patient on their side in case they vomit.

52. A. Hyperglycemia, or increased sugar in the blood, is common in type I diabetic patients. Other signs and symptoms include nausea and abdomen pain, weak pulse, and skin that is red and warm. Hypoglycemia, or decreased amount of sugar in blood, is common in type II diabetic patients. Signs and symptoms include rapid onset with dizziness, headache, poor coordination, hostile behavior, fainting, seizures, tachycardia, hunger, and skin that is cold, pale, and clammy.

53. B. Patients need a room with negative airflow (drawing air from hallway into room, out to outside, not recycled). In addition, a N95 mask should be fit to the individual.

54. A. Nosocomial infections are those acquired when in a healthcare facility.

55. C. Handwashing is the primary method of reducing infections.

56. D. Personal protection equipment used for transmission based precautions include gloves, gowns, and protective eyewear.

57. A. This is the most common way nosocomial (hospital acquired) infections are spread.

Suggested Readings

Bass LH, Anderson SL. Infection control in radiation oncology facilities. In: Washington CM, Leaver D, editors. Principles and practice of radiation therapy. 3rd ed. St. Louis, MO: Mosby Elsevier; 2010. p. 190–225.

Brant JM. Pain. In: Yarbro CH, Wujcik D, Gabel BH, editors. Cancer symptom management. 4th ed. Burlington, MA: Jones & Bartlett Learning; 2014. p. 69–92.

Callaghan M, Cooper A. Alopecia. In: Yarbro CH, Wujcik D, Gabel BH, editors. Cancer symptom management. 4th ed. Burlington, MA: Jones & Bartlett Learning; 2014. p. 495–506.

Coleman AM. Treatment procedures. In: Washington CM, Leaver D, editors. Principles and practice of radiation therapy. 3rd ed. St. Louis, MO: Mosby Elsevier; 2010. p. 158–79.

Cunningham RS. The cancer cachexia syndrome. In: Yarbro CH, Wujcik D, Gabel BH, editors. Cancer symptom management. 4th ed. Burlington, MA: Jones & Bartlett Learning; 2014. p. 351–84.

Dutton AG, Linn-Watson T, Torres LS. Torres' patient care in imaging technology. 8th ed. Baltimore, MD: Walters Kluwer Health; 2013.

Eatmon S. Cancer: an overview. In: Washington CM, Leaver D, editors. Principles and practice of radiation therapy. 3rd ed. St. Louis, MO: Mosby Elsevier; 2010. p. 3–21.

Krebs LU. Altered body image and sexual health. In: Yarbro CH, Wujcik D, Gabel BH, editors. Cancer symptom management. 4th ed. Burlington, MA: Jones & Bartlett Learning; 2014. p. 507–40.

Leaver D. Detection and diagnosis. In: Washington CM, Leaver D, editors. Principles and practice of radiation therapy. 3rd ed. St. Louis, MO: Mosby Elsevier; 2010. p. 86–102.

Maihoff SE, Dungey G. Patient assessment. In: Washington CM, Leaver D, editors. Principles and practice of radiation therapy. 3rd ed. St. Louis, MO: Mosby Elsevier; 2010. p. 226–46.

Mitchell SA. Cancer-related fatigue. In: Yarbro CH, Wujcik D, Gabel BH, editors. Cancer symptom management. 4th ed. Burlington, MA: Jones & Bartlett Learning; 2014. p. 27–44.

Morse L. Skin and nail bed changes. In: Yarbro CH, Wujcik D, Gabel BH, editors. Cancer symptom management. 4th ed. Burlington, MA: Jones & Bartlett Learning; 2014. p. 587–616.

Muehlbauer PM, Lopez RC. Diarrhea. In: Yarbro CH, Wujcik D, Gabel BH, editors. Cancer symptom management. 4th ed. Burlington, MA: Jones & Bartlett Learning; 2014. p. 185–212.

Tipton J. Nausea and vomiting. In: Yarbro CH, Wujcik D, Gabel BH, editors. Cancer symptom management. 4th ed. Burlington, MA: Jones & Bartlett Learning; 2014. p. 213–40.

Wilson B. Patient interactions. In: Adler A, Carlton R, editors. Radiologic sciences and patient care. 4th ed. St. Louis, MO: Saunders Elsevier; 2005. p. 141–56.

Wilson BG. The ethics and legal considerations of cancer management. In: Washington CM, Leaver D, editors. Principles and practice of radiation therapy. 3rd ed. St. Louis, MO: Mosby Elsevier; 2010. p. 22–43.

Yarbro CH, Berry DL. Bladder disturbances. In: Yarbro CH, Wujcik D, Gabel BH, editors. Cancer symptom management. 4th ed. Burlington, MA: Jones & Bartlett Learning; 2014. p. 265–84.

Chapter 9
Professional Issues

Questions

1. When must the radiation therapy prescription be signed by the radiation oncologist?

   A. Before the simulation
   B. Before the first treatment
   C. Before the fifth treatment
   D. Any time during the patient's course of treatment

2. Which of the following pieces of information is not required to be in the radiation therapy treatment prescription?

   A. Treatment site
   B. Total dose to be delivered
   C. Information describing treatment technique
   D. Beam angles

3. Daily patient identification may be completed by (Choose all correct answers):

   A. Patient ID wristband
   B. Asking patient to spell their last name
   C. Calling patient's first name
   D. Patient identification card or barcode

4. When using a paper chart to record radiation therapy treatments, the radiation therapist should:

   A. Use ink to record all aspects of treatment
   B. Use white out or correction tape if an error occurs
   C. Sign their name, as well as the radiation therapist they are working with that day
   D. All of the above are acceptable

© Springer Science+Business Media New York 2016

A. Heath, *Radiation Therapy Study Guide*, DOI 10.1007/978-1-4939-3258-0_9

5. Which of the following scenarios does not meet the definition of a radiation therapy medical event?

   A. Total dose differing by 5 % from the prescribed total dose
   B. Fraction dose exceeding prescribed fraction dose by 50 %
   C. Total dose differing by 30 % from the prescribed total dose
   D. All of the above are considered radiation therapy medical events

6. If a radiation therapy medical event is discovered, when must the NRC, or NRC designee, be verbally notified?

   A. Within 24 h of when the event occurred
   B. Within 24 h of when the event was discovered
   C. Within 15 working days of when the event occurred
   D. Within 15 working days of when the event was discovered

7. ICD Codes describe:

   A. Patient demographics
   B. Provider demographics
   C. Patient diagnosis
   D. Patient outcomes

8. Which of the following in not true regarding Current Procedural Terminology (CPT) codes?

   A. Published by the American Medical Association
   B. Coding system to describe procedures completed by physicians and other staff
   C. Composed of five letters
   D. Codes are updated annually

9. The process of agreeing to treatment, documented by patient signature, after learning of the risks, benefits, outcomes, and alternatives to a procedure is termed:

   A. Implied consent
   B. Informed consent
   C. Verbal consent
   D. Documented consent

10. Whose responsibility is it to obtain informed consent?

    A. Physician
    B. Nurse
    C. Radiation therapist
    D. Medical dosimetrist

11. In order to give consent, individuals must be:

    A. 18 years or older
    B. Emancipated minor
    C. Parent of child receiving care
    D. All of the above

12. Mary, a radiation therapist, noticed her neighbor's name on the simulator schedule. Outside of work, Mary asked her neighbor about her appointment, violating patient:

    A. Confidentiality
    B. Privacy
    C. Patient care
    D. Code of Conduct

13. Confidentiality is not guaranteed when:

    A. State law requires otherwise
    B. When the patient's life is in danger, or moral obligation to another is dictated
    C. A and B
    D. Confidentiality is always guaranteed

14. Patient privacy can be improved by:

    A. Covering patients when possible
    B. Allow patient to wear gowns or robes
    C. Leaving the room to allow patients to disrobe or dress
    D. All of the above

15. What end-of-life care or directive describes supportive care used for patients who have a life expectancy of less than 6 months?

    A. Palliative care
    B. Hospice care
    C. Do not resuscitate (DNR) order
    D. Living will

16. Personal injury laws are considered:

    A. Tort laws
    B. Criminal laws
    C. Contract laws
    D. Administrative laws

17. Using restraints without an order from a physician is considered:

    A. Libel
    B. Battery
    C. False imprisonment
    D. Slander

18. Providing care less than the standard level of care is termed:

    A. Assault
    B. Negligence
    C. Respondeat Superior
    D. Res Ipsa Loquitur

19. Which is not true regarding the ARRT Standard of Ethics:

    A. Intended for protection, safety, and comfort of patients
    B. Must be followed by registered radiologic technologists and radiation therapists
    C. Are not applicable for radiologic technologists and radiation therapists applying for certification by the ARRT
    D. Promote ethical behavior within the profession

20. The patient must be identified by the following number of methods prior to each daily treatment:

    A. 1
    B. 2
    C. 3
    D. 4

21. Who in the radiation oncology department is required to complete HIPAA training?

    A. Physicians, nurses, and radiation therapists
    B. All individuals who may be exposed to confidential information
    C. Physicians, nurses, radiation therapists, physicists
    D. Nurses, radiation therapists, physicists, front-desk staff

Answers and Rationales

1. B. The radiation therapy prescription is the order for radiation treatment. The prescription *must* be signed (signature and date) by the radiation oncologist prior to the administration of radiation treatment, *no exceptions*.
2. D. The following items must be included in the prescription: anatomic site, total radiation dose to be delivered, fractionation and protraction schedule, and treatment technique (the number and orientation of treatment fields). Other items commonly found in the radiation prescription: beam energy, portal sizes and entry angles, and beam modifiers.
3. A, C, and D. The treatment record must include a patient photograph for visual identification. Two methods of patient identification must be used on a daily basis to confirm patient identify prior to treatment administration. Methods of identification may include: identification cards presented by the patient, a bar-coding system (requires patient identification cards and an electronic charting system/patient management system), patient wristbands, and requesting the patient to state their birth date or spell last name.
4. A. Each entry in a patient record must be accompanied by the signature of the person who makes the entry. Each entry in a paper record must be made in ink. The signature must be clear so that it is evident who is participating in the patient's care. In electronic record, electronic signature is used from unique user names and passwords. When correcting an error in a paper record, the following steps should be taken:

   - Draw a single line through the incorrect entry.
   - Initial, time stamp and date the correction.
   - Record the correct information.
   - Never erase, black out, or cover up errors with correction fluid.

5. A. A radiation therapy (external beam) medical event is any of the following: the total dose delivered differs from the prescribed dose by 20 % or more, the fractionated dose delivered exceeds the prescribed dose, or a single fraction, by 50 % or more, an administration of a dose to the wrong patient, an administration of a dose delivered by the wrong mode of treatment.
6. B. The NRC should be notified by telephone within one calendar day of the discovery of the event. A written report should be provided within 15 days of the discovery.
7. C. International Classification of Disease (ICD) provides specific codes to describe diagnosis and treatment of medical services. Codes are constructed of numbers and letters, which correspond to specific illnesses, injuries, and procedures. They are required by CMS and private third-party payers to be included on every reimbursement claim. Coding allows patient-specific information to remain confidential.
8. C. Codes are composed of five numbers. They are divided into technical and professional categories.

9. B. Informed consent is the process in which an individual participates in his/her healthcare by agreeing to or refusing a treatment based on full disclosure of all treatment details (including but not limited to risks, benefits, probable outcome, and alternative options).

10. A. It is the physician's responsibility to obtain informed consent.

11. D. Patients must have legal capacity to give consent. Legal capacity is defined as 18 years of age or older and legally deemed competent, legal guardian of an incompetent adult, an emancipated minor (determined by the court), parent or legal guardian of a child, or an individual obligated by court order.

12. A. Medical and personal patient information a patient is strictly confidential, and only those involved in the patient's care should access the patient record. Patient information should never be shared with others outside the workplace.

13. C. Confidentiality is not guaranteed when state law requires otherwise or when the patient's life is in danger, or moral obligation to another is dictated. An example would be an emergency situation.

14. D. To maintain patient privacy, the radiation therapist should cover the patient as much as possible, allow a private area to change and/or disrobe, and provide gowns to cover patients while they are waiting for their treatment.

15. B. Palliative Care provides patients with relief from symptoms and/or pain with the goal of improving quality of life for the patient and their family. Hospice Care provides palliative and supportive care for patients with a life expectancy of less than 6 months in the patient's home or a hospice facility. Do Not Resuscitate (DNR) is a legal order to not undergo CPR or advanced cardiac life support if a patient's heart were to stop if patient stopped breathing. The request is made by either the patient or health care power of attorney. A Living Will is a document which indicates how the patient would like his/her care provided in the event that they become incompetent to make their own medical decisions.

16. A. Civil Law rules noncriminal activities. Tort law, a type of civil law, is personal injury law.

17. C. False imprisonment is intentional confinement without proper authorization. Another example is holding a patient against their will. Libel is written defamation of character, while slander is oral defamation of character. Battery is touching a patient without their consent.

18. B. Assault is the threat of touching in an injurious way. Respondeat Superior is the legal doctrine which states that employers are responsible for negligent acts by their employees while performing job duties. Res Ipsa Loquitur is latin for "the thing speaks for itself," meaning standards of practice serves as basis for what someone should or should not do.

19. C. ARRT Standard of Ethics provides guidance on what it means to be qualified, as well as promotes ethical behavior within the profession. These standards apply solely to persons holding certificates from ARRT, as well as those apply for certification by the ARRT. They consist of a *Code of Ethics* and *Rules of Ethics*. The Code of Ethics serves as a guide of professional conduct and is

intended to assist in maintaining a high level of ethical conduct and in providing for the protection, safety, and comfort of patients. The Rules of Ethics outlines the mandatory standards of minimally acceptable professional conduct for all Certificate Holders and Candidates.

20. B. Patients must be identified through two methods each day for treatment. Examples may include: having patients spell their last name, provide their date of birth, inpatient wristband, and face photo.

21. B. Any person who has access to patient information must undergo annual HIPAA training in order to maintain compliance.

Suggested Readings

American Medical Association. 2013 Current procedural terminology—professional edition. 2012.

ARRT standard of ethics. The American Registry of Radiologic Technologists.2013. https://www.arrt.org/pdfs/Governing-Documents/Standards-of-Ethics.pdf. Accessed 15 Feb 2013.

Chapter DHS 157. Wisconsin Legislative, Documents. https://docs.legis.wisconsin.gov/code/admin_code/dhs/157/VIII/83.

Coleman AM. Treatment procedures. In: Washington CM, Leaver D, editors. Principles and practice of radiation therapy. 3rd ed. St. Louis: Mosby Elsevier; 2010. p. 158–79.

Wilson B. The ethics and legal considerations of cancer management. In: Washington CM, Leaver D, editors. Principles and practice of radiation therapy. 3rd ed. St. Louis: Mosby Elsevier; 2010. p. 22–43.

Chapter 10
Review of Pathophysiology

Questions

1. A change in the size, shape, and organization of a cell is defined as:

    A. Hypertrophy
    B. Hyperplasia
    C. Metaplasia
    D. Dysplasia

2. Neoplasia is:

    A. Increase in size of cell
    B. Abnormal, rapid growth of benign or malignant cells
    C. Decrease in size and function of a cell
    D. Change in number of cells in a tissue

3. Which is not a sign of inflammation?

    A. Coolness of tissue
    B. Edema
    C. Pain
    D. Loss of function

4. Swelling in tissue caused by excessive extravascular fluid is termed:

    A. Sepsis
    B. Edema
    C. Hematoma
    D. Extravasation

© Springer Science+Business Media New York 2016
A. Heath, *Radiation Therapy Study Guide*, DOI 10.1007/978-1-4939-3258-0_10

5. A blood clot passing through a vessel with the ability to obstruct the lumen of a vessel is termed:

   A. Thrombus
   B. Embolism
   C. Infarction
   D. All of the above are correct

6. Thrombocytopenia characterizes a decreased number of:

   A. Platelets
   B. Formed elements of blood (RBCs, WBCs, and platelets)
   C. White blood cells
   D. Red blood cells

7. Which is not a risk factor for hypertension?

   A. Older age
   B. Smoking
   C. High-fiber diet
   D. Family history

8. An epidural hematoma is when there is a hematoma between:

   A. Skull and dura mater
   B. Dura mater and arachnoid mater
   C. Arachnoid mater and pia mater
   D. Pia mater and brain

9. What disease of the central nervous system is characterized by progressive demyelinization of neurons, with plaque formation around the nerves?

   A. Multiple sclerosis
   B. Alzheimer's disease
   C. Schizophrenia
   D. Meningitis

10. A cataract of the eye is:

    A. Increased pressure within the eye
    B. Clouding of the lens of the eye
    C. Central impairment of the vision field
    D. Inflammation of the conjunctiva

11. The eye disorder that involves increased pressure within the eye is called

    A. Cataract
    B. Glaucoma
    C. Macular degeneration
    D. Retinal detachment

12. What is the medical term used for a middle-ear infection?

    A. Presbycusis
    B. Otitis media
    C. Acoustic otitis
    D. Presbyotitis

13. Which of the following is not a sign or symptom of hyperthyroidism?

    A. Increased metabolism
    B. Exopthalmus
    C. Decreased blood pressure
    D. Anxiety

14. Which of the following is true regarding hypothyroidism?

    A. Patients present with weight gain
    B. More common in men
    C. Treated with radioactive iodine
    D. Caused by overabundance of thyroid hormones

15. What term is used to describe enlargement of male breasts due to proliferation of glandular tissue?

    A. Fibrocystic breasts
    B. Fibroadenoma
    C. Gynecomastia
    D. Breast cancer

16. The most common benign breast tumor is:

    A. Fibrocystic breasts
    B. DCIS
    C. Fibroadenoma
    D. Gynecomastia

17. Air in the pleural cavity is referred to as:

    A. Atelectasis
    B. Pneumothorax
    C. Pleural effusion
    D. Pneumonia

18. What is the name of the condition that results in fluid accumulating in the pleural space?

    A. Pleuritis
    B. Pleural effusion
    C. Pulmonary embolism
    D. Pneumothorax

19. Inflammation and consolidation of the pulmonary parenchyma describes

    A. Lung abscess
    B. Adult respiratory distress syndrome
    C. Pneumoconiosis
    D. Pneumonia

20. What disorder is characterized by the stomach contents backing into the esophagus?

    A. Gastroesophageal reflux disorder (GERD)
    B. Barrett's esophagus
    C. Peptic ulcer disease
    D. Crohn's disease

21. Which of the following is not true regarding type 1 diabetes?

    A. Common in children
    B. Pancreas does not produce insulin
    C. Can be managed by diet and exercised
    D. Rapid onset of symptoms

22. Abdominal weight gain, moon face, buffalo hump, and hypertension are all signs and symptoms of what endocrine disorder?

    A. Addison's disease
    B. Cushing's syndrome
    C. Acromegaly
    D. Pancreatitis

23. What strain of hepatitis is spread through contaminated food and water?

    A. Hepatitis A
    B. Hepatitis B
    C. Hepatitis C
    D. All of the above

24. Which is not true regarding jaundice?

    A. Results in yellowed skin and sclera
    B. Caused by increased destruction of RBC's
    C. Caused by obstruction of bile
    D. Uncommon in newborns

25. A urinary tract infection of the kidney is termed:

    A. Nephrolithiasis
    B. Pyelonephritis
    C. Cystitis
    D. Urethritis

26. What disorder of the male reproductive system results in nocturia, polyuria and decreased pressure of the urinary system?

    A. Cryptorchidism
    B. Phimosis
    C. Benign prostatic hypertrophy
    D. All of the above

27. The presence of endometrial tissue outside of the uterus, which engorges and sheds in a cyclic manner like the menstrual cycle is termed:

    A. Uterine fibroids
    B. Endometriosis
    C. Ovarian cysts
    D. Polycystic ovarian syndrome

28. A sign or symptom of polycystic ovarian syndrome is:

    A. Amenorrhea
    B. Ascites
    C. Vaginal discharge
    D. Polyuria

29. Risk factors for osteoporosis include all of the following except:

    A. Late menopause
    B. Family history
    C. Small build
    D. Smoking

30. The most common joint disease is:

    A. Osteoarthritis
    B. Rheumatoid arthritis
    C. Atherosclerosis
    D. Osteoporosis

31. The medical term for hives is:

    A. Dermatitis
    B. Urticaria
    C. Psoriasis
    D. Scleroderma

32. Fungal infections (Choose all that apply):

    A. Occur in skin folds
    B. Cause itching
    C. Are treated with antibiotics

33. The inflammatory skin condition that involves a very increased rate of cellular proliferation is:

    A. Scleroderma
    B. Psoriasis
    C. Eczema
    D. Lichen planus

Answers and Rationales

1. D. Hypertrophy is an increase in size and function of a cell. Hyperplasia is an increase in the number of cells in an organ or tissue. Metaplasia is transformation of the cell into a different cell type, and dysplasia is a change in the size, shape, and organization of cell.
2. B. Hypertrophy is an increase in size and function of a cell, atrophy is decrease in size and function of a cell, and dysplasia is a change in the size, shape, and organization of cell.
3. A. Inflammation is a nonspecific defense that occurs in response to tissue injury in order to prepare tissue for healing. The five signs of inflammation include redness, heat, edema, pain, and loss of function.
4. B
5. B. A blood clot inside the lumen of a blood vessel and fixed to the blood vessel wall is termed a thrombus. An embolism is a blood clot not fixed to blood vessel wall, but is rather passing through the blood vessel with the ability to obstruct the lumen of the vessel. An infarction can occur in any blood vessel causing ischemic necrosis in nearby tissue and is caused by blood clot obstructing the blood vessel.
6. A. Pancytopenia describes a decreased number of formed elements (RBCs, WBCs, platelets) in the blood, while thrombocytopenia is a decreased number of platelets.
7. C. The risk of hypertension or a chronic elevation of blood pressure ($\geq$140/90 mm Hg), is increased due to: advanced age, family history, genetic factors, obesity, diabetes, smoking, and alcohol abuse. Consequences of hypertension are kidney damage, stroke, aneurysms, congestive heart failure, and atherosclerosis.
8. A. There are four types of intracranial hemorrhages. Epidural hematoma occur between skull and dura mater, and must be treated quickly and aggressively to prevent coma and death. Subdural hematomas are between arachnoid and dura mater, and are often a result of a blow to the head affecting venous blood flow which stops quickly and requires little to no treatment. A subarachnoid hematoma occurs between arachnoid and brain surface, often due to a ruptured congenital aneurysm or trauma. Finally, an intracerebral hematoma results from trauma which ruptures the intracerebral vessels causing bleeding into the brain. It can be caused by high blood pressure, leading to a stroke or by blood disorders which clot the blood.
9. A. Multiple sclerosis (MS) is a progressive demyelinization of neurons, with plaque formation around the nerves. There is a higher incidence of MS in colder climates and in women, involving a series of flare-ups and remissions with progressive loss of motor and sensory function. Alzheimer's disease is the most common cause of dementia, causing generalized atrophy of brain with plaques and neurofibrillary tangles. Schizophrenia is characterized by psychotic symptoms that significantly impair functioning and that involve disturbances in feeling, thinking, and behavior. Meningitis is inflammation of the brain and

spinal cord often caused by viral or bacterial infections, resulting in pus in the cerebrospinal fluid (CSF). Signs and symptoms include: fever, headache, lethargy, stiff neck, confusion, and irritability.

10. B.

11. B. Glaucoma is increased pressure within the eye damaging the optic nerve, causing blindness. Macular degeneration results in central impairment of the vision field, while peripheral vision remains normal. Conjunctivitis, or pink eye, is inflammation of the conjunctiva due to virus, bacteria, or allergens.

12. B. Presbycusis describes age-related hearing loss, while otitis media refers to a middle-ear infection due to bacteria or a virus resulting in pain and pressure. Otitis media is commonly resolved with antibiotics.

13. C. Hyperthyroidism is very common in women, caused by an overproduction of thyroid hormones. Signs and symptoms include: faster metabolism resulting in weight loss, feeling warm and intolerance to heat, increased appetite, increased heart rate and blood pressure, anxiety, menstrual changes, and exophthalmos. Hyperthyroidism is treated with radioactive iodine.

14. A. Hypothyroidism is also very common in women, caused by thyroid hormone deficiency. Signs and symptoms include slowed metabolism, fatigue, difficulty concentrating, feeling cold, slowed heart rate, weight gain, and constipation. Hypothyroidism is treated with oral thyroid medication.

15. C.

16. C. Fibrocystic breasts are a cystic dilatation of terminal ducts in the breasts, resulting in an increase in fibrous tissue, which can be painful. Fibroadenoma is the most common benign breast tumor, characterized by a round, movable, rubbery feeling mass.

17. B.

18. B.

19. D. Atelectasis describes a lung collapse due to obstruction or compression. Pneumothorax is air in pleural cavity. Pneumonia is inflammation and consolidation of pulmonary parenchyma. COPD (chronic obstructive pulmonary disease) is another common lung disorder, resulting in chronic airway obstruction due to chronic bronchitis and/or emphysema. Chronic bronchitis results in permanent damage to bronchi of the lung and is often caused by smoking. With emphysema, the alveolar walls are damaged, resulting in poor gas exchange, over-inflated lungs, and a barrel chest.

20. A. GERD is a disorder in which the stomach contents back up into esophagus through lower esophageal sphincter (LES). This causes pain, burning and discomfort. Barrett's esophagus can be caused by chronic GERD, in which the squamous epithelium is replaced by columnar epithelium. Peptic ulcer disease, or gastric ulcers are created when there are breaks in the gastric mucosa from gastric secretions. Crohn's disease is inflammation of all five layers of bowel wall, causing edema and fibrosis of the bowel. This results in a decreased lumen and the potential for bowel obstruction, malabsorption, and malnutrition, and high risk for intestinal cancer.

21. C. Type 1 diabetes is caused by autoantibodies, mostly in childhood and adolescence, causing the pancreas to produce little to no insulin. Type 1 diabetes

presents with a rapid onset of symptoms, and requires the patient to intake insulin by mouth or injection. Type 2 diabetes is caused by insulin resistance and insulin deficiency, and is most common in obese adults. Some cases of type 2 diabetes can be managed with diet restrictions and exercise, but others may require diabetic medications and insulin.

22. B. Addison's disease is an adrenal insufficiency due to destructive atrophy of the adrenal glands caused by long term use or sudden withdrawal of oral steroids. Signs and symptoms include: weakness, hypotension, hypoglycemia, weight loss, and hyperpigmentation. Cushing's syndrome can be caused by a pituitary tumor (Cushing's disease), small cell lung cancer secretion of ACTH, or steroids. Signs and symptoms include abdominal weight gain, moon face (round face), buffalo hump (fat pad on upper back), thinning skin, purple striae (stretch marks) on abdomen, thighs, and arms, hirsutism, mood swings, insomnia, loss of libido, hypertension, and osteoporosis.

23. A. Hepatitis A is spread via oral-fecal route by improper hand-washing or contaminated food and water. It is often asymptomatic or may cause "flu-like" symptoms and resolve itself. Hepatitis B and C are spread via bodily fluids.

24. D. Jaundice is caused by high levels of circulating bilirubin, by-product of breakdown of RBCs, resulting in yellowed skin and sclera. While common in newborns, jaundice may also be caused by liver disease, metastatic cancer in the liver, or obstruction of bile flow.

25. B. Nephrolithiasis, or kidney stones, are calcium stones in the kidney due to high levels of circulating calcium. Urinary tract infections can occur anywhere along urinary tract. A kidney infection is termed pyelonephritis, a bladder infection is termed cystitis and an infection in the urethra is termed urethritis.

26. C. Cryptorchidism, or undescended testicle, present at birth and may resolve itself in first year of life or need surgery to bring down. Cryptorhidism results in an increased risk of infertility, and increased risk of developing testicular cancer. Phimosis, or inability to retract foreskin of penis, may be congenital or due to infection or inflammation. Benign prostatic hypertrophy (BPH) is enlargement of prostate causing obstruction of urinary flow, causing nocturia, polyuria, and decreased pressure of urinary stream, hesitancy, and dribbling. Treatment for BPH is medication or surgery.

27. C.

28. A. Signs and symptoms of endometriosis include dysmenorrhea, pain with intercourse (dyspareunia), and fallopian tube damage. Uterine fibroids are benign tumors of the myometrium, which are often asymptomatic. If the fibroids are large enough, they can cause pain, pressure on the bladder or rectum, and heavy menstrual bleeding. Ovarian cysts are a common cause of pelvic pain and typically do not require treatment. Polycystic ovarian syndrome (PCOS) are enlarged ovaries with multiple cysts. The ovaries do not function normally, usually no ovulation (infertile). Signs and symptoms include amenorrhea or very infrequent menses, excess androgen hormones, causing hirsutism and obesity. Patients with PCOS are at increased risk of diabetes and endometrial cancer because of

hormone abnormalities. Treatment is prescription of birth control pills, in order to create normal hormonal cycles.

29. A. Osteoporosis is a reduction in bone density over time, causing fragile bones and fractures. Risk factors include family history, thin or small build, fair skin, early menopause, past age 50, smoking, sedentary lifestyle, and inadequate dietary calcium or vitamin D. Complications of osteoporosis include hip or vertebral fractures and chronic pain.

30. A. Osteoarthritis, or wear and tear arthritis, is the most common joint disease. Rheumatoid arthritis is a chronic systemic, autoimmune disease involving synovial joints, causing extreme deformities of the knuckles, wrists, elbows, and ankles.

31. B. Urticaria, or hives, is an allergic reaction due to a histamine release. Treatment is antihistamines, or epinephrine in severe cases. Dermatitis, or inflammation of the skin, results in red, swollen and itchy skin. Psoriasis results in increased rates of skin sloughing and growth causing thickening of the dermis and epidermis. Treatment for psoriasis are steroids and UV light. Scleroderma is a collection of collagen deposits in the skin causing inflammation, fibrosis, and decreased capillary networks.

32. A and B. Fungal infections tend to occur in warm, dark, and moist environments such as under the breasts or abdomen, in skin folds, on scalp, feet, groin, and diapered area of young children. Fungal infections also cause itching, scaling, and sometimes burning. Treatment is either topical or oral antifungal agents.

33. B.

Suggested Readings

McConnell TH. The nature of disease: pathology for the health professions. Baltimore, MD: Lippincott, Williams, and Wilkins; 2007.

Chapter 11
Clinical Components of Cancer Care

Questions

1. Which of the following is true regarding the epidemiology of cancer?

    A. Risk increases with increased age
    B. Caucasians have a higher incidence of cancer than African Americans
    C. Women have a higher incidence of cancer than men
    D. Men and women develop the same types of cancer equally

2. An example of a carcinogen classified as a physical agent is:

    A. Smoke
    B. Nitrates
    C. Viruses
    D. Asbestos

3. An example of an iatrogenic risk factor for cancer is:

    A. BRCA 1 gene
    B. Working in the petroleum industry
    C. Prior chemotherapy
    D. Diet high in fat

4. Li-Fraumeni syndrome is an example of a _____ risk factor for cancer.

    A. Occupational
    B. Virus
    C. Genetic
    D. Diet

© Springer Science+Business Media New York 2016
A. Heath, *Radiation Therapy Study Guide*, DOI 10.1007/978-1-4939-3258-0_11

5. Incidence refers to:

   A. The number of new cases of a disease in a particular time period
   B. The number of deaths from a disease in a particular time period
   C. Duration of time from diagnosis to death
   D. Number of individuals with a disease at a specific point in time

6. Women should have annual mammograms after the age of:

   A. 30
   B. 35
   C. 40
   D. 45

7. A sign is:

   A. A test which has the ability to give a true positive
   B. Subjective indication of disease as reported by the patient
   C. A test which has the ability to give a true negative
   D. Objective finding found by the examiner

8. After the age of 50, colonoscopies should be completed every _____ years.

   A. 2
   B. 5
   C. 10
   D. 15

9. Tumor marker CA 19–9 aids in the diagnosis of:

   A. Breast cancer
   B. Colorectal cancer
   C. Prostate cancer
   D. Ovarian cancer

10. What imaging study is best for soft tissue visualization?

    A. Radiographs
    B. MRI
    C. Nuclear medicine
    D. CT Scan

11. A _____ is a malignant tumor of connective tissue.

    A. Lipoma
    B. Adenocarcinoma
    C. Squamous cell carcinoma
    D. Sarcoma

12. Which of the following is a characteristic of benign tumors?

    A. Encapsulated
    B. Grow quickly
    C. Spread through lymphatics
    D. Are destructive to the host

13. A Grade 2 tumor is:

    A. Undifferentiated
    B. Poorly differentiated
    C. Moderately differentiated
    D. Well differentiated

14. Gleason scores are used with what type of cancer?

    A. Breast
    B. Prostate
    C. Head and Neck
    D. Cervical

15. The presence of metastatic disease is indicated in which part of the TNM stage?

    A. T
    B. N
    C. M
    D. All parts of the TNM staging system

16. What staging system is used for lymphomas?

    A. FIGO System
    B. Ann Arbor Staging
    C. Duke's Staging
    D. Kaplan–Meier System

17. Concurrent treatment:

    A. Follows the primary treatment
    B. Is given at the same time as another treatment
    C. Occurs before another treatment
    D. A and C

18. Which type of biopsy would be useful to obtain cells from a cystic tumor?

    A. Fine needle aspiration
    B. Core needle biopsy
    C. Excisional biopsy
    D. Wedge biopsy

19. An example of a patient who is inoperable is a patient with a/an:

    A. Tumor adjacent to the heart
    B. Pre-existing health condition
    C. Tumor on the face
    D. Tumor where it would be difficult to obtain negative margins

20. Chemotherapy is less concentrated when administered through _____ methods.

    A. Oral
    B. Intravenous
    C. Intracavitary
    D. Intrarterial

21. Adriamyacin is toxic to the:

    A. Lung
    B. Colon
    C. Heart
    D. Brain

22. Gemcitabine is what type of chemotherapy drug?

    A. Alkylating
    B. Platinum based
    C. Plant Alkaloid
    D. Antimetabolite

23. Brachytherapy treatment to the breast is an example of:

    A. Intracavitary brachytherapy
    B. Surface brachytherapy
    C. Interstitial brachytherapy
    D. Intralumen brachytherapy

24. An example of prophylactic external beam radiation is:

    A. Whole brain treatment for small cell lung cancer
    B. Stereotactic radiation to single brain metastasis
    C. Whole brain treatment in a patient with symptomatic disease
    D. Conformal treatment to a primary brain tumor

25. What is true regarding preoperative chemotherapy or radiation therapy?

    A. Uses higher doses than when used alone
    B. Used to treat microscopic disease
    C. Are used to increase resectability of tumor in surgery
    D. Is never used, is only indicated postoperatively

Answers and Rationales

1. A. Factors that affect epidemiology of cancer include age (in general, incidence increases with age), gender (women have lower incidence and higher survival; men and women also develop different types of cancer), ethnicity/race (overall, African-Americans have a higher incidence of cancer than Caucasians), and environment/ geography (varies by regions within a country, or by countries themselves).
2. D. Carcinogens may be chemical (tar, smoke, food additives, insecticides), physical agents (ionizing radiation, asbestos, chronic trauma), or viruses, infections, hormones, and diet.
3. C. Iatrogenic risk factors are those caused by treatment to a medical condition. Chemotherapy and radiation therapy are both iatrogenic risk factors for cancer.
4. C. Risk factors may be environmental (pollution, sun exposure), occupational (farmers, leather workers, tanners, petroleum workers), viruses (Ebstein-Barr virus, Human papilloma virus, Hepatitis B virus), genetics (BRCA 1, BRCA2, Li-Fraumeni syndrome, Familial adenomatous polyposis), lifestyle (smoking and tobacco use, alcohol consumption), diet (high in fat, low in fiber) or iatrogenic (prior chemotherapy or radiation therapy).
5. A. Incidence refers to the number of new cases in a period of time in a defined population. Survival is the duration of time from diagnosis to death, while prevalence refers to the number of individuals with a given disease in a given population during a specified period of time. Mortality is the number of deaths attributed to cancer in a specified time period and in a defined population.
6. C. American Cancer Society recommends women should have annual mammograms after the age of 40; clinical breast exams every 3 years after the age of 20 in addition to monthly self-breast exams.
7. D. Signs are objective finding (can be seen, touched, etc.) found by the examiner, while symptoms are subjective indication of disease as reported by the patient. Tests with the ability to give a true positive are sensitive tests, while tests with the ability to give a true negative are specific tests.
8. C. After the age of 50, flexible sigmoidoscopy should be completed every 5 years, a barium enema every 5 years and a colonoscopy every 10 years.
9. B. Common tumor markers are outlined in Table 11.1.
10. B. In Computed Axial Tomography, or a CT Scan, the x-ray beam rotates 360°, lined up to a specific plane in the body. Sensors on the outside of the CT receive

Table 11.1 Common tumor markers used in the diagnosis of cancer

Tumor marker	Cancer types
CEA: Carcinoembryonic antigen	Colon and breast cancer
AFP: Alphafetoprotein	Liver, testicular, pancreatic, and gastric tumors
HCG: Human chorionic gonadotrophin	Germ cell tumors, seminomas
Acid phosphatase	Prostate
PSA: Prostate specific antigen	Prostate
CA 19–9	Colorectal
CA-125	Ovarian

messages and create a picture. MRI, or Magnetic Resonance Imaging, uses a magnetic force rather than radiation exposure and is good for soft tissue visualization. Gadolinium is used as contrast, and no metal or pacemakers are allowed near the scanner. Ultrasound uses high frequency sound waves. A transducer makes and sends sound waves, which bounce off structure and back to the transducer. Mammography is used to detect breast cancers, and can tell calcifications vs. tumor. With Nuclear Medicine scans, the patient is injected with a radionuclide. The radionuclide gets stuck at site of involvement, and gamma cameras pick up radionuclides that are being emitted.

11. D. A benign tumor of fatty tissue is termed a lipoma. Malignant tumors of epithelial cells are carcinoma (adenocarcinoma is a malignant tumor of glandular cells, while squamous cell carcinomas are malignant tumors of squamous cells). Sarcomas are malignant tumors in connective tissue: bone (osteosarcoma), muscle (leimyosarcoma and rhabdomyosarcoma) and, cartilage (chondrosarcoma).

12. A. Benign tumors tend to stay localized, though can grow in size slowly. They are encapsulated, are well-differentiated, and typically have little effect on normal tissue or host. Malignant tumors invade locally, as well as distantly as they metastasize through lymphatic spread, hematologous spread and seeding. These tumors can grow quickly and infiltrate outside of capsule. Malignant tumors can be destructive to normal tissue and host, and vary from well differentiated to undifferentiated (depending on grade of tumor).

13. C. Grading measures how differentiated a cell is, thus provides information regarding aggressiveness of tumor. Grade 1 is well differentiated, Grade 2 is moderately differentiated, Grade 3 is poorly differentiated, and Grade 4 is undifferentiated.

14. B. Gleason score is a specific grading system used in prostate cancer.

15. C. Staging is determined by the patient care team after a complete work-up has been completed and measures extent of tumor and disease spread. Staging may be clinical (from information gathered in the diagnostic process) or surgical (from information gathered in the surgical process). In the TNM system, the letters indicate:

   A. T—Size and extent of primary tumor, typically indicated by 1–4, higher stage indicates larger size or extent of tumor.
   B. N—Involvement of lymph nodes, typically indicated by 1–4, higher stage indicates increased involvement of lymph nodes.
   C. M—Presence of metastatic disease, typically indicated by 0 (no metastatic disease), 1 (metastatic disease present), or x (metastatic disease not assessed).

16. B. The FIGO system is used for gynecological malignancies, Ann Arbor Staging system is used for lymphomas and Duke's Staging is used for colorectal tumors.

17. B. Many patients receive multimodality treatment to manage their cancer. Primary treatment describes when one treatment primarily used. Neoadjuvant treatment is when one treatment given prior to the other, while adjuvant treatment means in addition to and may follow another treatment. Concurrent treatments are given at the same time, typically on the same day.

18. A. Surgical biopsies are used for diagnostic purposes. Fine needle biopsy uses a small gauge needle and removes fluid or cells. Core needle biopsy uses a large gauge needle and removes a tissue specimen. Excisional biopsies removes the entire lesion as one specimen.

19. B. Not all patients are surgical candidates. Patients may be inoperable— pre-existing health conditions prohibits them from withstanding anesthesia required for the surgery- or unresectable— tumor is located close to normal structures, would be difficult to get negative margins or would leave cosmetic defect.

20. D. Chemotherapy can be administered in variety of modalities, dependent on drug and cancer type. Oral administration is easiest for patients to administer themselves. Intravenous is the most common method, and intracavitary is used for bladder cancers. With intraarterial administration, drugs are less concentrated in this delivery. Other methods include intrathecal and injections. Patients often have PICC lines or ports placed for administration of chemotherapy agents.

21. C. See Table 11.2 for classification, agents, clinical use and toxicities.

Table 11.2 Common chemotherapy agents

Type of agent	Drugs	Clinical use	Toxicity	How it works
Alkylating agents	Cychlophosphamide	Lymphoma	Hematological (decreases blood counts)	Inhibits DNA synthesis
	Nitrogen mustard	Breast cancer	Infertility	
Platinum based alkylating agents	Cisplatin	Head and neck, cervix, lung, bladder	Hematological, renal, neurological (deafness)	Cross links DNA
	Carboplatin			
Antimetabolites	5-FU	Colorectal	Hematological	Imitates DNA building blocks
	Gemcitabine	Lymphoma	GI Symptoms	
	Methotrexate	Breast	Skin toxicities	
Topoisomerase I Inhibitors	Topothecan	Breast	Hematological	Blocks enzymes involved in DNA transcription and replication
	Irinotecan	Lymphoma	Cardiac	
		Sarcoma		
Plant alkaloids	Taxotere	Breast	Hematologic	Interferes with mitosis, destroys microtubule mechanism
	Taxol	Lung	Neurologic	
	Vincristine	Testicular	Alopecia	
	Etopóside			
Antitumor antibiotics	Adriamyacin	Leukemia	Adriamyacin— cardiac	Interferes with DNA and RNA transcription
	(Doxorubicin) Actinomyocin D	Lymphoma	Bleomycin— lung	
	Bleomycin	GI		
Hormones	Tamoxifen	Breast	Can mimic menopause symptoms	Block hormone receptors or eliminate hormones
	Arimidex	Prostate		
	Lupron			
	Zoladex			

22. D. See Table 11.2 for classification, agents, clinical use and toxicities.
23. C. Brachytherapy delivers dose quickly with excellent fall off of dose. With interstitial brachytherapy, sources are placed in tissue. Sources placed in a cavity is termed intracavitary brachytherapy and when placed in a tubular structure, it is termed interluminary brachytherapy.
24. A. Radiation therapy can be used for cure, control, palliation or prophylactic (whole brain for small cell lung cancer metastasis).
25. C. Preoperative radiation therapy or chemotherapy is often used to shrink the tumor to increase its resectability; lower doses are often used. Postoperative radiation therapy or chemotherapy is used to treat microscopic disease, or tumor left after surgery; clips are often left in surgery to identify tumor location.

Suggested Readings

Bussman-Yeakel L. Digestive system tumors. In: Washington CM, Leaver D, editors. Principles and practice of radiation therapy. 3rd ed. St. Louis, MO: Mosby Elsevier; 2010. p. 764–802.

Choy H, MacRae R, Story M. Basic concepts of chemotherapy and irradiation interaction. In: Halperin EC, Perez CA, Brady LW, editors. Principles and practice of radiation oncology. 5th ed. Philadelphia, PA: Lippincott Williams & Wilkins; 2008. p. 669–88.

Eatmon S. Cancer: an overview. In: Washington CM, Leaver D, editors. Principles and practice of radiation therapy. 3rd ed. St. Louis, MO: Mosby Elsevier; 2010. p. 3–21.

Giordano PJ. Principles of pathology. In: Washington CM, Leaver D, editors. Principles and practice of radiation therapy. 3rd ed. St. Louis, MO: Mosby Elsevier; 2010. p. 44–56.

Green S. Lymphoreticular system tumors. In: Washington CM, Leaver D, editors. Principles and practice of radiation therapy. 3rd ed. St. Louis, MO: Mosby Elsevier; 2010. p. 610–28.

Kuban DA, Trad ML. Male reproductive and genitourinary tumors. In: Washington CM, Leaver D, editors. Principles and practice of radiation therapy. 3rd ed. St. Louis, MO: Mosby Elsevier; 2010. p. 823–65.

Leaver D. Detection and diagnosis. In: Washington CM, Leaver D, editors. Principles and practice of radiation therapy. 3rd ed. St. Louis, MO: Mosby Elsevier; 2010. p. 86–102.

Milas L, Cox JD. Principles of combining radiation therapy and chemotherapy. In: Cox JD, Ang KK, editors. Radiation oncology. Rational, technique, results. 8th ed. St. Louis, MO: Mosby Elsevier; 2003. p. 108–24.

Zagars GK. Principles of combining radiation therapy and surgery. In: Cox JD, Ang KK, editors. Radiation oncology. Rational, technique, results. 8th ed. St. Louis, MO: Mosby Elsevier; 2003. p. 97–107.

Chapter 12
Cancers of the Brain and Central Nervous System

Questions

1. The _____ lobe of the brain has a role in a person's personality.

   A. Frontal
   B. Parietal
   C. Temporal
   D. Occipital

2. What lobe in the cerebrum is the most posterior?

   A. Frontal
   B. Parietal
   C. Temporal
   D. Occipital

3. On CT scan, the texture of this structure resembles that of cauliflower, and is gray in color.

   A. Frontal lobe
   B. Cerebellum
   C. Hypothalamus
   D. Pituitary gland

4. The most inferior portion of the brain stem is:

   A. Medulla oblongata
   B. Midbrain
   C. Pons
   D. Spinal cord

© Springer Science+Business Media New York 2016
A. Heath, *Radiation Therapy Study Guide*, DOI 10.1007/978-1-4939-3258-0_12

5. What structure in the brain is (are) horn shaped?

A. Pons
B. Lateral ventricles
C. Cerebral aquaduct
D. Infundibulum

6. What covering of the brain is closest to the skull?

A. Arachnoid mater
B. Dura mater
C. Pia mater
D. Epi mater

7. What extension of the dura mater separates the cerebellum from the cerebrum?

A. Falx cerebelli
B. Falx cerebri
C. Tentorium cerebelli
D. Tentorium cerebri

8. Cerebrospinal fluid is contained within the _____ space.

A. Subdural
B. Subarachnoid
C. Epidural
D. Arachnoid

9. The cribiform plate is a structure of this bone:

A. Frontal
B. Ethmoid
C. Sphenoid
D. Parietal

10. This bone contains the dorsum sellae:

A. Sphenoid
B. Occipital
C. Temporal
D. Frontal

11. What structure within the brain is responsible for supplying arterial blood to the cerebrum?

A. Thalamus
B. Corpus callosum
C. Hypothalamus
D. Circle of Willis

12. At what vertebral level does the spinal cord end?

    A. T12
    B. L2
    C. L4
    D. S2

13. Adult tumors in the central nervous systems are typically located:

    A. In the spinal cord
    B. In the brain stem
    C. Supratentorial
    D. Infratentorial

14. What is the most common age of diagnosis for malignant gliomas?

    A. 35–45 years old
    B. 45–55 years old
    C. 55–65 years old
    D. 65–75 years old

15. Patients with a tumor in the cerebrum may present with any of the following signs and symptoms except:

    A. Headaches
    B. Visual changes
    C. Deferred pain in the thorax
    D. Nausea and vomiting

16. The preferred imaging modality for the diagnosis of brain tumors is:

    A. MRI
    B. CT
    C. PET
    D. Radiographs

17. The most common malignancy in the brain is:

    A. Astrocytoma
    B. Glioma
    C. Metastatic disease
    D. Oligodendroglioma

18. Ependymomas typically spread via:

    A. Lymphatic spread
    B. Seeding through the CSF
    C. Invasion into the cerebellum
    D. Extension through base of skull

19. Which of the following may be included in a patient's treatment plan for a glioblastoma multiforme? Choose all correct answers.

    A. Temozolomide
    B. External beam radiation therapy
    C. Surgery
    D. Interferon
    E. Corticosteroids

20. Margins of _____ are typically added to the tumor and edema when planning 3D conformal radiation therapy for a primary brain tumor.

    A. 0.5 cm
    B. 2 cm
    C. 4 cm
    D. 6 cm

21. Simulation for patients with brain tumors would include immobilization via:

    A. Thermoplastic immobilization device
    B. Vacuum bag immobilization device
    C. Chemical mold
    D. Abdominal compression

22. Which of the following is not a common chronic effect of external beam radiation to the brain?

    A. Alopecia
    B. Necrosis
    C. Vision changes
    D. Headache

23. What is the inferior border of the spine field when treating a patient with craniospinal irradiation (CSI)?

    A. C2
    B. T12
    C. L2
    D. S2

24. Glioblastoma multiforme has a prognosis of:

    A. Less than 1 month
    B. Less than 1 year
    C. 5 years
    D. Almost always curable

Answers and Rationales

1. A. The cerebrum is the largest and most superior part of brain, divided into right and left halves, and located superior to the tentorium. The cerebrum is comprised of four lobes (two of which are paired): frontal (1), parietal (2), temporal (2), and occipital (1). The frontal lobe is anterior and superior, responsible for muscle control, speech, and personality. Parietal lobes are located at top of head, and responsible for sensory functions. Temporal lobes are located inferior to parietal lobes, and responsible for auditory functions. Finally, the occipital lobe is posterior, and responsible for visual functions.

2. D. See Question 1 for details about the different parts of the brain.

3. B. The cerebellum is the second largest part of brain and located inferior to the tentorium. The function of the cerebellum is to control skeletal muscles, which maintains balance, controls posture and coordination. On CT scan, the cerebellum sits posterior and inferior within the skull, has cauliflower-like texture, and is gray in appearance.

4. A. The brain stem consists of midbrain, pons, and medulla oblongata and connects the brain to the spinal cord. The most superior portion of the brain stem is the midbrain, next is the pons, and finally the medulla oblongata is the most inferior portion. On CT scan, the brain stem is seen centrally within the brain just superior to the foramen magnum.

5. B. The ventricles are large, fluid filled cavities within the brain. There are four of them. The lateral ventricles (2) are horn like structures within the cerebrum lined with ependymal cells, which form the choroid plexus. The choroid plexus produces cerebrospinal fluid (CSF). On CT scan, one can see the lateral ventricles through several slices; it sits midline in the cerebrum and is dark gray in color. The third ventricle is inferior to anterior horn of lateral ventricle. CSF travels from lateral ventricles here and is produced here as well. The fourth ventricle is a triangular shaped structure, and receives CSF from the third ventricle through the cerebral aqueduct. On CT scan, the fourth ventricle is located anterior to the cerebellum.

6. B. The dura mater is closest to the skull. Next, is the arachnoid mater. This middle layer is delicate and cobweb like in nature. Finally, the pia mater is closest to the brain and contains blood vessels.

7. C. Falx cerebri is the extension of dura mater which separates two hemispheres of the cerebrum. The falx cerebelli is the extension of dura mater which separates two hemispheres of the cerebellum. The tentorium cerebelli is the extension of dura mater which separates the cerebellum from the cerebrum.

8. B. Spaces between the meninges include the epidural space, subdural space and subarachnoid space. The epidural space is located between the dura mater and the bone covering of the brain and spinal cord. The subdural space is located between the dura mater and arachnoid membrane and contains lubricating fluid. The subarachnoid space is located between the arachnoid and pia mater and contains cerebrospinal fluid.

9. B. The frontal bone forms the forehead, anterior skull and roofs of orbital cavities. Parietal bones make up the lateral wall and roof of skull. The sphenoid bone is considered the floor of the cranium, and articulates with all cranial bones. The sphenoid bone contains the sphenoid sinus, dorsum sellae and hypophyseal fossa. The ethmoid bone contains the crista galli and cribriform plate. The paired temporal bones forms inferior portion of the lateral wall of the cranium and the middle cranial floor, and contains the mastoid air cells and external auditory meatus. Finally, the occipital bone forms the posterior aspect of skull, and forms the foramen magnum.

10. A. See Question 9 for details about the bones of the skull.

11. D. The Circle of Willis is a structure which contains vessels that supply arterial blood to the cerebrum. The corpus callosum are large bundles of white matter which connect the left and right cerebral hemispheres. The thalamus forms the lateral walls of the third ventricle, and serves role in sensory impulses. The hypothalamus forms the floor and walls of the third ventricle, and serves an important role in homeostasis.

12. B. The spinal cord extends from the foramen magnum to L2. The spinal cord contains white and gray matter. The outer layer of the cord is white matter, and nerve fibers are located here. The inner core of grey matter contains the nerve cells. The spinal cord receives impulses from the body and transmits to the brain, as well as sends signals back to the body from the brain through 31 pairs of spinal nerves.

13. C. Adult brain tumors are located superior to the tentorium, while pediatric brain tumors are located inferior to the tentorium.

14. B. There are an estimated 22,000 cases of CNS malignancies per year and 13,000 deaths. The most common age for diagnosis of malignant gliomas is 45–55 years old and 30–40 years old for low-grade gliomas. The cause is mostly unknown, though there are several occupational, environmental, and lifestyle causes thought to be linked.

15. C. Patients present with headaches, seizures, nausea, and vomiting, regardless of tumor location (often due to increased intracranial pressure). Location of the tumor can cause specific symptoms as well. Frontal lobe tumors can present with personality changes, temporal lobe tumors may present with aphasia, dementia, memory impairment, personality changes, and parietal lobe tumors will present with sensory changes.

16. A. Diagnostic exams include a CT of the head, followed by MRI to obtain detailed information regarding the size and extension of the tumor. Gadolinium is used for contrast for the MRI procedure. Images should be T1 and T2 weighted (T2 weighted shows edema). H & P should include examination of coordination, motor and sensory skills, eye exam (papilledema would indicate increased intracranial pressure), and neurologic work-up (mental and intellectual status, speech, memory and logic). A PET scan may be used to determine necrosis vs. tumor.

17. C. Metastatic disease is the most common malignancy of the brain. In regards to primary brain tumors, 82 % of primary brain tumors are astrocytomas, anaplastic astrocytomas, or glioblastoma multiforme. Other histologies include

medulloblastoma, oligodendrocytoma, mixed oligoastrocytoma, ependymomas, and meningiomas. Primary brain tumors are classified by the WHO grading system (I–IV), based on cell origin and how the cells behave.

18. B. Direct, local extension is primary pathway for spread of most primary brain tumors. Medulloblastomas and ependymomas seed through the CSF.

19. A, B, C, and E. Patients are usually prescribed dexamethasone to manage intracranial pressure. Surgery is primary treatment for primary brain tumors, but even gross total resection does not typically remove all cancerous cells so post-operative radiation therapy is typically given. Post-operative radiation is the mainstay of treatment and can be delivered to the CNS by fractionated external beam, radiosurgery, stereotactic irradiation, or brachytherapy. Chemotherapy is not standard of care, but newer drugs that can cross the blood–brain barrier have been shown to be useful in certain types of cancers. Temozolomide is currently being used in some clinical situations.

20. B. Radiation therapy is delivered 2–4 weeks after surgery to allow for wound healing. Fields are planned using 3D conformal treatment, treating GTV (tumor and edema) with 2 cm margins. Vertex fields and wedge pairs are common field arrangements. The fields are given a total dose of 45–60 Gy in 1.8–2.0 Gy fractions, and may include a cone-down boost at 50 Gy.

21. A. Patients are positioned supine, with the head positioned in thermoplastic masks for immobilization. If treating with craniospinal fields, patients may be treated in the prone position.

22. D. Organs at risk when treating tumors within the brain include the lens of the eye, optic nerve, optic chiasm, normal brain, brainstem, spinal cord, pituitary gland. Acute toxicities of radiation therapy to the brain include fatigue, hair loss, and skin erythema. Late toxicities include brain necrosis, L'Hermitte's syndrome, somnolence, lethargy and chronic headaches.

23. D. If disease has spread into the CSF, craniospinal irradiation (CSI) may be used, typically matching whole brain and spine fields. Depending on the patient's height, two spine fields may need to use two fields (superior and inferior) and match on skin. The inferior border of the spine field is placed at the bottom of S2 to ensure treatment of all space in which CSF flows.

24. B. Prognosis of primary brain tumors are affected by age (increased age decreases survival), histology and grade, and patient performance status. Five-year survival rates for primary gliomas are 29–35 %.

Suggested Readings

Adams RD, Leaver D. Central nervous system tumors. In: Washington CM, Leaver D, editors. Principles and practice of radiation therapy. 3rd ed. St. Louis, MO: Mosby Elsevier; 2010. p. 745–63.

Madden M. Introduction of sectional anatomy. 2nd ed. Baltimore, MD: Wolters Kluwer-Lippincott Williams and Wilkins; 2008.

Shah AA. Management of adult central nervous system tumors. In: Chao KSC, Perez CA, Brady LW, editors. Radiation oncology management decisions. 3rd ed. Philidelphia, PA: Wolters Kluwer-Lippincott Williams and Wilkins; 2011. p. 145–92.

Stockham AL, Suh JH, Chao ST. Central nervous system radiotherapy. In: Videtic GMM, Vassil AD, editors. Handbook of treatment planning in radiation oncology. New York, NY: Demos Medical Publishing; 2011. p. 25–40.

Thibodeau G, Patton K. Anatomy and physiology. 5th ed. St. Louis, MO: Mosby-Elsevier; 2003.

Vann A, Dasher BG, Wiggers NH, Chesnut SK. Portal design in radiation therapy. 3rd ed. Augusta, GA: DWV Enterprises; 2013.

Chapter 13
Cancers of the Head and Neck Region

Questions

1. What structure in the head and neck is anterior to the nasopharynx?

   A. Nasal cavity
   B. Pharynx
   C. Cervical spine
   D. Parotid glands

2. The retromolar trigone is a structure in this cavity in the head and neck:

   A. Nasopharynx
   B. Oropharynx
   C. Oral cavity
   D. Nasal cavity

3. The pharyngeal tonsils are located within the:

   A. Nasopharynx
   B. Oropharynx
   C. Hypopharynx
   D. Nasal cavity

4. The true vocal cords are located within the:

   A. Pyriform sinuses
   B. Supraglottis
   C. Glottis
   D. Subglottis

5. What vertebral body is also known as the axis?

 A. C1
 B. C2
 C. C7
 D. T3

6. The hyoid bone is located at what vertebral body?

 A. C1
 B. C3
 C. C5
 D. C7

7. Stenson's ducts transport saliva from the _____ glands.

 A. Submandibular
 B. Sublingual
 C. Parotid
 D. Submaxillary

8. Which of the following is true regarding the lymphatics of the head and neck?

 A. Submental nodes are inferior to the body of the mandible
 B. Cervical nodes are superficial only
 C. Retropharyngeal node is the primary lymph node in the head and neck
 D. Lymphatics may be labeled by groups, chains, or levels

9. Which is true regarding the epidemiology of head and neck cancer?

 A. More common in males than females
 B. Most common cancer in males
 C. Common in patients in the 20s
 D. Cancer of the oropharynx is the most common

10. Which is not a risk factor for head and neck cancer?

 A. Smoking
 B. Alcohol use
 C. HPV
 D. Obesity

11. Which is not a common sign or symptom of head and neck cancer?

 A. Hoarseness
 B. Migraine headaches
 C. Trismus
 D. Dysphagia

12. What diagnostic exam for head and neck cancer involves the use of a light and mirror to visualize structures?

    A. Indirect laryngoscopy
    B. Swallow study
    C. Direct laryngoscopy
    D. MRI

13. The most common histology of head and neck cancer is:

    A. Squamous cell carcinoma
    B. Adenoid cystic carcinoma
    C. Adenocarcinoma
    D. Melanoma

14. Nasopharyngeal tumors spread to the _____ nodes.

    A. Submental
    B. Anterior cervical
    C. Retropharyngeal
    D. Facial

15. What surgery removes lymph nodes, the sternocleidomastoid muscle on one or both sides, cranial nerve 11, as well as regional soft tissue?

    A. En bloc resection
    B. Radical neck dissection
    C. Extraction
    D. Decompression surgery

16. Which of the following is true regarding external beam radiation to the head and neck region? Choose all correct answers.

    A. Will include tumor and regional lymphatics
    B. Treat to a total dose of 50 Gy
    C. May treat with IMRT
    D. May treat with shrinking field technique
    E. Concurrent chemotherapy is not used

17. Positioning and immobilization for head and neck treatment may include all of the following except:

    A. Respiratory gating
    B. Thermoplastic immobilization devices
    C. Removal of dentures
    D. Shoulder assistance straps

18. If treating a patient with conformal radiation, what structure would you limit dose to primarily?

    A. Parotid gland
    B. Oral mucosa
    C. Vocal cord
    D. Thyroid cartilage

19. Acute side effects of external beam radiation therapy to the head and neck include all of the following except:

    A. Esophagitis
    B. Erythema
    C. Mucositis
    D. Trismus

20. Treatment to cancers of the true glottis would include:

    A. Radiation therapy to the vocal cords only
    B. Comprehensive radiation therapy to larynx and draining lymphatics
    C. Radical neck dissection
    D. Concurrent chemotherapy and radiation therapy

Answers and Rationale

1. A. The nasal cavity is located superior to the hard palate and oral cavity, and anterior to the nasophyarnx. The function of the nasal cavity is to transport, filter, and warm air, as well as help with resonance of voice.

2. C. The oral cavity is located inferior to the nasal cavity and anterior to the oropharynx. Structures within the oral cavity include the interior surface of the lips, gingiva, buccal mucosa, retromolar trigone, hard palate, floor of mouth, and anterior 2/3 of the tongue. On CT scan, the oral tongue is prominent, surrounded by the aveolar ridge of the mandible and maxilla.

3. A. The pharyngeal tonsils are located within the nasopharynx, which is located posterior to nasal cavity and inferior to base of skull. The palatine and lingual tonsils are located within the oropharynx, as well as the uvula and vallecula. The superior border of the oropharynx is the nasopharynx, while the anterior border is the junction of soft and hard palate, and the inferior border is at the level of the hyoid bone. On CT scan, the oropharynx will often be black as it is air filled.

4. C. The larynx is located between the hyoid bone and cricoid bone, and has three subdivisions. The supraglottis is the most superior subdivision and contains the false cords, aryepiglottic folds and arytenoids. The glottis contains the true vocal cords, while the subglottis is the most inferior subdivision.

   The hypopharynx surrounds the laryngeal tube and contains the posterior pharyngeal wall and pyriform sinuses.

5. B. There are seven vertebrae of the cervical spine, which have foramina in their transverse processes which vertebral arteries pass through to the brain. C1, or the atlas, is located near inferior margin of the nasopharynx. C2, or the axis, has a dens which projects superior to serve as body of C1. C7 has a very long spinous process, or vertebral prominence.

6. B. The hyoid bone is a "U"-shaped bone floating bone located at the level of C3. On CT scan, this U-shaped bone surrounds the pharynx, and is inferior to body of the mandible. The thyroid cartilage is located below the hyoid bone at the level of C4. The cricoid cartilage is circular in shape and surrounds the pharynx inferior to the thyroid cartilage.

7. C. The bilateral submandibular glands are inferior to the mandible. Saliva formed in these ducts enter the digestive system through Wharton ducts. On CT scan, these glands are lateral to the hyoid bone, identifiable by noted difference in texture from surrounding soft tissues. The bilateral parotid glands are lateral to the rami of the mandible, anterior to the ear. Saliva formed in the parotid glans enter digestive system through Stenson's ducts. On CT scan, these glands are anterior to the ear and lateral to the rami of the mandible, identifiable by noted difference in texture from surrounding soft tissues. The sublingual glands are the numerous salivary glands located inferior to the oral tongue.

8. D. The lymphatics in the head and neck may be labeled by groups, chains or levels. Submandibular nodes are located inferior to the body of the mandible

(level 1) and submental nodes are located inferior to tip of chin (level 1). The cervical chain may be divided into superficial or deep, based upon location in respect to the sternocleidomastoid muscle. The jugulodigastric nodes are located at angle of mandible and are the primary lymph node of the head and neck.

9. A. Head and neck cancers represent 3-8% of all cancers in the United States and is more common in males than females. Nasopharyngeal cancer incidence is high in patients of Asian or Chinese descent. Cancer of the larynx has the highest incidence of all head and neck cancers.

10. D. Risk factors for head and neck cancer include smoking and smokeless tobacco use, alcohol consumption, Epstein-Barr virus (nasopharynx), HPV (oropharynx), and history of leukoplakia (oral cancer).

11. B. Signs and symptoms of head and neck cancer include ulceration, hoarseness, lump in the neck, dysphagia, otalgia, trismus, and epitaxsis.

12. A. An indirect laryngoscopy uses a light and mirror to visualize structures of the pharynx, while a direct laryngoscopy uses a fiber-optic scope. Other diagnostic exams used in head and neck cancer include H&P, CT, MRI, swallow study, and dental evaluation.

13. A. Squamous cell carcinoma is the most common histology of head and neck cancer.

14. C. Primary lymphatic involvement is the jugulodigastric node and cervical chains (levels 2 and 3). Tip of tongue lesions drain to submental nodes, while nasopharynx tumors drain to retropharyngeal nodes. The true glottis has no lymphatic drainage. Head and neck cancers also spread directly through local invasion into surrounding structures (bone, cartilage, nerves, muscles, blood vessels).

15. B. Radical neck dissection is used for some head and neck cancers. Nasopharynx cancers cannot be surgically removed due to their location; radiation therapy is primary treatment for this subtype.

16. A, C, and D. IMRT is used now to decrease the dose to sensitive structures and decrease long-term toxicities, with the nodal volume receiving 50–54 Gy and the target GTV dose receiving 70–74 Gy. Traditionally, a shrinking field technique was used. The large lateral fields would use low energy photons to treat the tumor and all regional lymphatics, shrinking at 40–45 Gy to just include tumor and anterior lymph nodes. Posterior lymph nodes were treated with posterior electron strip fields in order to limit the dose to the spinal cord. This field was matched to the photon fields anteriorly. Anterior lateral fields would shrink to boost just the GTV to a total dose of 72–75 Gy. An anterior supraclavicular field would also be used to treat the supraclavicular lymph nodes to a dose of 54 Gy, matching lateral neck fields daily. Cisplatin or carbo-platin chemotherapy is used concomitantly with radiation therapy.

17. A. Patients are immobilized using thermoplastic masks. A bite block or similar device may be used to keep jaw in same position each day, as well as push the tongue or hard palate out of the way for treatment. If the patient has dentures,

these should be removed for simulation and treatment. Shoulder assistance straps may be used to pull the shoulders out of treatment for the lateral fields.

18. A. Organs at risk when treating head and neck cancer include the parotid glands, lens, ear, spinal cord, mucous membranes, brain, larynx, thyroid, mandible, esophagus, and temporomandibular joint. Treatment of the parotid glands result in the most troublesome and common late effect, xerostomia. The use of hyper-fractionation may be used to decrease long-term toxicities.

19. D. Acute side effects include fatigue, skin reactions, mucositis, dysphagia, and tissue necrosis. Late effects include xerostomia (#1), hoarseness, trismus, alopecia, dental caries, and osteoradionecrosis of the mandible.

20. A. As the true glottis has no lymphatics, radiation therapy to the vocal cords only would be used for treatment. Vocal cord stripping or laser surgery are also treatment options.

Suggested Readings

Burri RJ. Nasopharynx. In: Chao KSC, Perez CA, Brady LW, editors. Radiation oncology management decisions. 3rd ed. Philadelphia, PA: Wolters Kluwer-Lippincott Williams and Wilkins; 2011. p. 211–26.

Koyfman SA, Greskovich JH, Chao ST. Head and neck radiotherapy. In: Videtic GMM, Vassil AD, editors. Handbook of treatment planning in radiation oncology. New York, NY: Demos Medical Publishing; 2011. p. 41–66.

Lozano R. Head and neck cancers. In: Washington CM, Leaver D, editors. Principles and practice of radiation therapy. 3rd ed. St. Louis, MO: Mosby Elsevier; 2010. p. 692–744.

Madden M. Introduction of sectional anatomy. 2nd ed. Baltimore, MD: Wolters Kluwer-Lippincott Williams and Wilkins; 2008.

Parashar B. Oral cavity. In: Chao KSC, Perez CA, Brady LW, editors. Radiation oncology management decisions. 3rd ed. Philadelphia, PA: Wolters Kluwer-Lippincott Williams and Wilkins; 2011. p. 247–59.

Thibodeau G, Patton K. Anatomy and Physiology. 5th ed. St. Louis, MO: Mosby- Elsevier; 2003.

Vann A, Dasher BG, Wiggers NH, Chesnut SK. Portal design in radiation therapy. 3rd ed. Augusta, GA: DWV Enterprises; 2013.

Washingon CM. Surface and sectional anatomy. In: Washington CM, Leaver D, editors. Principles and practice of radiation therapy. 3rd ed. St. Louis, MO: Mosby Elsevier; 2010. p. 376–415.

Chapter 14
Cancers of the Respiratory System

Questions

1. What is not true regarding the trachea?

   A. Located between C1–T4
   B. Is C-shaped
   C. Located anterior to the esophagus
   D. Composed of cartilage

2. The most inferior portion of the lung is the:

   A. Apex
   B. Base
   C. Hilum
   D. Fissure

3. What vertebral level corresponds with the carina?

   A. T2–T3
   B. T4–T5
   C. T6–T7
   D. T8–T9

4. What chamber of the heart receives oxygenated blood from the pulmonary veins?

   A. Right atrium
   B. Right ventricle
   C. Left atrium
   D. Left ventricle

© Springer Science+Business Media New York 2016
A. Heath, *Radiation Therapy Study Guide*, DOI 10.1007/978-1-4939-3258-0_14

5. What is not a branch of the aorta?

   A. Axillary artery
   B. Brachiocephalic artery
   C. Common carotid artery
   D. Left subclavian artery

6. What portion of the sternum do the clavicles articulate with?

   A. Corocoid process
   B. Acromian process
   C. Manubrium
   D. Xiphoid

7. There are ___ pairs of floating ribs.

   A. 2
   B. 4
   C. 7
   D. 12

8. What is true regarding lymphatics of the thorax?

   A. Spread is predictable
   B. Interpulmonary nodes are located within the lung
   C. Mediastinal nodes are located between the left and right lung
   D. Lymphatics are sparse

9. Mesothelioma is linked to what risk factor?

   A. Asbestos exposure
   B. Smoking
   C. Radon
   D. Air pollution

10. The most common sign or symptom of lung cancer is:

   A. Hemoptysis
   B. Persistent cough
   C. Hoarseness
   D. Dyspnea

11. Which of the following procedures is not typically used for the work-up of lung cancer?

   A. Chest radiograph
   B. CT of the chest
   C. MRI of the chest
   D. Sputum cytology

12. Which histology is commonly linked with smoking and second-hand smoke?

    A. Mesothelioma
    B. Small-cell lung cancer
    C. Large-cell carcinoma
    D. Squamous cell carcinoma

13. A Pancoast tumor is located in what part of the lung?

    A. Apex
    B. Base
    C. Hilum
    D. Periphery

14. Which of the following is not a method of lung cancer spread?

    A. Direct into lung and ribs
    B. Distant to brain and liver
    C. Distant to colon
    D. Hilar and mediastinal lymph nodes

15. Which chemotherapy agent may be used in conjunction with radiation therapy to the lung?

    A. Platinum-based agent
    B. Herceptin
    C. Bleomyacin
    D. Avastin

16. Which is a contraindication of SBRT for lung cancer?

    A. Small, well-defined tumor
    B. Poor kidney function
    C. Small-cell histology
    D. Non-small-cell histology

17. Which of the following is not true regarding prophylactic cranial irradiation?

    A. Treat to total dose of 45 Gy
    B. Commonly used in patients with small-cell lung cancer
    C. Treated with whole-brain fields
    D. May cause temporary alopecia

18. External beam radiation to the lung typically begins with AP/PA fields, followed by oblique fields beginning at a dose of:

    A. 30 Gy
    B. 45 Gy
    C. 55 Gy
    D. 65 Gy

19. Acute side effects of radiation therapy to the lung include all of the following except:

    A. Pneumonitis
    B. Erythema
    C. Esophagitis
    D. Brachial plexopathy

20. Which of the following is not a prognostic factor for lung cancer?

    A. Weight loss
    B. KPS
    C. HPV status
    D. Histology

Answers and Rationales

1. A. The trachea is a C-shaped cartilage that connects the larynx and main bronchi, and is located from C6–T4. It sits anterior to the esophagus. On CT scan, the trachea is a midline structure that sits superior and anterior to the esophagus.

2. B. The apex is the most superior portion of the lung, while the base is the most inferior portion of the lung. The hilum is the central area of the lung where vessels and lymphatics are located. Lungs are divided into lobes which are separated by fissures. There are three lobes in the right lung and two lobes in the left lung.

3. B. The trachea enters the lungs and bifurcates into two main stem bronchi (this area is termed the carina and is at vertebral level T4–T5). The bronchi travel to each lung, and further divide to each lobe, segment, etc. The bronchi terminate into structures called aveoli. These small sacs, which are surrounded by blood vessels, are where gas exchange takes place.

4. C. There are four chambers of the heart. The right atrium collects venous, deoxygenated blood from the body via the inferior vena cava and superior vena cava. The right ventricle receives blood from the right atrium, sending it to the lungs by way of the pulmonary arteries. The left atrium collects arterial, oxygenated blood from pulmonary veins. The left ventricle receives blood from the left atrium and sends oxygenated blood to the body through aorta.

5. A. The aorta is the largest artery in the body, and originates from the left ventricle. The aorta is divided into thoracic (provides blood to organs above the diaphragm) and abdominal (provides blood to organs below the diaphragm). The thoracic aorta has three parts — ascending, arch of the aorta, and descending. The arch of the aorta is located at vertebral bodies T2–T3. The three major branches of the aorta are the brachiocephalic artery, left common carotid artery, and left subclavian artery. The aorta becomes the abdominal aorta once it enters the abdominal cavity and then birfurcates at the vertebral level of L4.

6. C. Bilateral clavicles connect with the acromian of the scapula and the manubrium of the sternum. The manubrium of the sternum is the superior portion, and also articulates with the first rib. The manubrium meets the body of the sternum inferiorly at the sternal angle or Angle of Louis. The body of the sternum, the middle section, articulates with ribs 2–10 directly or by costal cartilage. The inferior section is the xiphoid, which is located at vertebral level T10.

7. A. There are 12 pairs of ribs, which protect the thorax cavity. The true ribs (ribs 1–7), articulate with the sternum. The false ribs (ribs 8–10) articulate with the sternum indirectly via costal cartilage. Ribs 11–12 are the floating ribs, as they do not articulate with the sternum.

8. C. Because the constant movement of the lungs and heart, flow of the lymphatics in the thorax is unpredictable. Lymph nodes are identified by groups — mediastinal nodes (located in the mediastinum between the left and right lung) and intrapulmonary nodes (located within the lung).

9. A. Risk factors for lung cancer include smoking (including second hand smoke exposure), asbestos (mesothelioma), radon and air pollution.

10. B. Persistent cough is the most presentation of lung cancer. Other signs and symptoms may include hemoptysis, dyspnea, chest pain, hypercalcemia (SCLC), hoarseness (tumor pressing on recurrent laryngeal nerve), Horner's syndrome, and superior vena cava syndrome.
11. C. Diagnostic tests for lung cancer include chest radiographs, CT and PET scans, pulmonary function tests, sputum cytology, bone scans, and MRI of the brain.
12. B. Small-cell lung cancer (SCLC), or oat cell carcinoma, is associated with smoking. SCLC are typically centrally located tumors and are very aggressive. They are defined as limited or extensive stage.
13. A. Non-small-cell lung cancer (NSCLC) may be many histologies. Adenocarcinoma tumors are located in the periphery of lung. A Pancoast tumor is located in apex or superior sulcus of the lung. Squamous cell carcinomas are centrally located tumors. Other histologies may be large-cell or carcinoid tumors. Mesothelioma tumors are located in the pleural linings of the lung.
14. C. Lung cancer may spread through direct route to the lung, ribs, and spine, or through the lymphatic vessels to the hilar, mediastinal, and supraclavicular lymph nodes. Distantly, lung cancer spreads to the brain (especially SCLC), liver, bone, and adrenal gland.
15. A. SCLC is treated with combination radiation therapy and chemotherapy and is very sensitive to chemotherapy. Taxol and platinum-based chemotherapy is used.
16. C. Treatment for NSCLC is surgery if possible. If the patient is inoperable, SBRT is indicated.
17. A. Prophylactic cranial irradiation may be used for SCLC, to a total dose of 25–40 Gy.
18. B. Traditionally, AP/PA fields were used to treat lung cancer to a dose of 40–45 Gy, followed by off-cord oblique fields to a total dose of 65–70 Gy. Wedges were used to compensate for the slope of the chest. Now, tumors are treated with IMRT, SBRT or arc radiation therapy. Respiratory gating or abdominal compression may be used for motion management. Organs at risk are the lung, heart, cord, brachial plexus, esophagus, and ribs.
19. D. Acute toxicities of radiation therapy to the chest are skin toxicities, fatigue, esophagitis, and pneumonitis. Late toxicities include pneumonitis, brachial plexopathy, and rib fractures.
20. C. Prognostic factors include weight loss, KPS, stage, and histology. NSCLC has a 15–20 % 5-year overall survival, while SCLC has a 10–15 % 3-year overall survival.

Suggested Readings

Hunter GK, Videtic GMM. Thoracic radiotherapy. In: Videtic GMM, Vassil AD, editors. Handbook of treatment planning in radiation oncology. New York, NY: Demos Medical Publishing; 2011. p. 85–100.
Madden M. Introduction of sectional anatomy. 2nd ed. Baltimore, MD: Wolters Kluwer-Lippincott Williams and Wilkins; 2008.

Shah AA. Lung. In: Chao KSC, Perez CA, Brady LW, editors. Radiation oncology management decisions. 3rd ed. Philidelphia, PA: Wolters Kluwer-Lippincott Williams and Wilkins; 2011. p. 327–56.

Stinson D, Wallner PE. Respiratory system tumors. In: Washington CM, Leaver D, editors. Principles and practice of radiation therapy. 3rd ed. St. Louis, MO: Mosby Elsevier; 2010. p. 666–91.

Thibodeau G, Patton K. Anatomy and Physiology. 5th ed. St. Louis, MO: Mosby- Elsevier; 2003.

Vann A, Dasher BG, Wiggers NH, Chesnut SK. Portal design in radiation therapy. 3rd ed. Augusta, GA: DWV Enterprises; 2013.

Chapter 15
Cancers of the Digestive System

Questions

1. What is the innermost layer of the alimentary tract?

   A. Muscular
   B. Submucosal
   C. Serosal
   D. Mucosal

2. The upper esophagus drains to the _____ lymph nodes.

   A. Mediastinal
   B. Celiac
   C. Cervical
   D. Gastric

3. The stomach is located in which quadrant of the abdomen?

   A. Upper right
   B. Upper left
   C. Lower right
   D. Lower left

4. What structure within the small bowel increases the surface area in order to increase absorptions?

   A. Villi
   B. Rugae
   C. Peyer's patches
   D. Haustra

© Springer Science+Business Media New York 2016
A. Heath, *Radiation Therapy Study Guide*, DOI 10.1007/978-1-4939-3258-0_15

5. What section of the small bowel is closest to the stomach?

   A. Jejunum
   B. Duodenum
   C. Veriform appendix
   D. Ilium

6. What part of the large intestine runs horizontally across the abdominal cavity?

   A. Ascending colon
   B. Descending colon
   C. Sigmoid colon
   D. Transverse colon

7. Bile is secreted from this organ:

   A. Gallbladder
   B. Liver
   C. Pancreas
   D. Large intestine

8. The head of the pancreas sits near the:

   A. Spleen
   B. Jejunum
   C. Duodenum
   D. Hepatic flexure of the colon

9. What is not true regarding the epidemiology and etiology of esophageal cancer?

   A. More common in those 55 years old and older
   B. Primary risk factor is smoking and alcohol
   C. More common in females
   D. Barrett's esophagus is a risk factor

10. What histology is common in tumors of the upper two-thirds of the esophagus?

    A. Adenocarcinoma
    B. Papillary serous carcinoma
    C. Squamous cell carcinoma
    D. Transitional cell carcinoma

11. Lymphatic drainage of the esophagus:

    A. Is predictable
    B. Skips up to 5 cm from the tumor site
    C. Is contiguous
    D. Is uncommon

12. What is a late toxicity of radiation therapy to the esophagus?

    A. Myelosuppression
    B. Stenosis
    C. Fatigue
    D. Esophagitis

13. Which of the following is not a risk factor for stomach cancer?

    A. Smoked, cured food
    B. Low socioeconomic status
    C. *H. pylori*
    D. GERD

14. What histology are most stomach cancers?

    A. Adenocarcinoma
    B. Papillary serous carcinoma
    C. Squamous cell carcinoma
    D. Transitional cell carcinoma

15. What is the primary treatment for cancer of the stomach?

    A. Immunotherapy
    B. Radiation therapy
    C. Chemotherapy
    D. Surgery

16. What site is the most common cancer in the GI system?

    A. Esophagus
    B. Stomach
    C. Pancreas
    D. Colon

17. Risk factors for colorectal cancer includes all of the following except:

    A. Plummer Vinson syndrome
    B. Diet high in fat, low in fiber
    C. History of polyps
    D. Smoking

18. Which of the following does not aid in the diagnosis of colorectal cancer?

    A. Colonoscopy
    B. Fecal occult blood test
    C. Ultrasound
    D. CT

19. What staging system is used with colorectal cancer?

    A. Ann Arbor
    B. FIGO
    C. Duke's
    D. Clarke's

20. Which beam arrangement is most commonly used for rectal cancer?

    A. Four-field pelvis, patient supine
    B. Four-field pelvis, patient prone
    C. Three-field pelvis, patient prone
    D. Three-field pelvis, patient supine

21. Anal carcinoma are typically what histology?

    A. Squamous cell carcinoma
    B. Adenocarcinoma
    C. Mucoid carcinoma
    D. Transitional cell carcinoma

22. What is not a sign or symptom of anal cancer?

    A. Rectal bleeding
    B. Pain
    C. Small bowel obstruction
    D. Anal mass

23. What is the primary lymphatic drainage of anal cancer?

    A. Superficial inguinal nodes
    B. Common iliac nodes
    C. Para-aortic nodes
    D. Pre-sacral nodes

24. What is not a risk factor for pancreatic cancer?

    A. Smoking
    B. Chronic pancreatitis
    C. Diabetes
    D. High-fiber diet

25. Patients presenting with jaundice most likely have pancreatic tumors in the
    ____ of the pancreas.

    A. Periphery
    B. Head
    C. Body
    D. Tail

26. What tumor marker is used with pancreatic cancers?

    A. CEA
    B. CA 19-9
    C. AFP
    D. PSA

27. Primary treatment for pancreatic cancer is:

    A. Whipple surgery
    B. Chemotherapy
    C. IMRT radiation therapy
    D. Observation

28. The 5-year overall survival of pancreatic cancer is:

    A. 100 %
    B. 60 %
    C. 30 %
    D. <10 %

Answers and Rationales

1. D. The alimentary tract has four layers (from inner to outer): mucosal, submucosal (contains blood vessels and lymphatics), muscular, and serosal (attaches to peritoneum).
2. C. The esophagus is a collapsible tube which transports food to stomach, extending from the mouth to the stomach. It sits posterior to the trachea and anterior to the spinal bodies between C6 and T10–11. The upper esophagus drains to the cervical, deep jugular and supraclavicular lymph nodes, while the middle esophagus drains to the supraclavicular and mediastinal lymph nodes and the proximal esophagus drains to the mediastinal and celiac lymph nodes. On CT scan the esophagus sits medial in the body between the trachea and cervical spine and upper thoracic spine; it shifts to the left as it meets with the stomach. The esophagus is difficult to visualize without contrast.
3. B. The stomach is located in upper left quadrant of the abdomen between T10–L3, and connects esophagus and small bowel. Major structural components of the stomach include the fundus (superior portion), body (middle portion), pyloris (inferior portion), cardiac sphincter (sphincter located between the esophagus and fundus of stomach), and pyloric sphincter (sphincter located between the pylorus of the stomach and duodenum). On CT scan, the stomach is visualized in the abdominal cavity of the left side of the body. The fundus of the stomach is anterior to the spleen. As you scan inferiorly, the stomach will move anterior and inferior. At the pyloris, the stomach is anterior to the pancreas.
4. A. The small bowel connects the stomach with the large intestine. Villi, located in the mucosal layer, increase surface area of the small bowel to increase absorption. Peyer's patches are aggregates of lymphoid tissue in the small bowel. Haustra are pouches within colon, which help move waste through the colon.
5. B. The duodenum is the superior portion of the small bowel, and connects the pyloris of the stomach with jejunum. It is C shaped and surrounds the head of the pancreas. The jejunum connects the duodenum and ilium, and most of the digestion takes place here. The ilium is the inferior portion of the small bowel, and connects jejunum and cecum of large intestine. On CT scan, small bowel loops throughout the abdominal cavity (typically midline), and is smaller in diameter than the large intestine.
6. D. The large intestine begins with the cecum. The cecum is located in lower right quadrant. Next, the ascending colon is on right side of abdominal cavity, running from the cecum to the hepatic flexure of colon. The transverse colon runs horizontally across abdominal cavity between hepatic and splenic flexures, and is inferior to liver, stomach, and spleen. The descending colon is on the left side of abdomen, between the splenic flexure and sigmoid colon. The curved sigmoid colon connects the descending colon and rectum. Next the rectum connects the sigmoid colon with anus, which is the end of the alimentary tract. On CT scan, the large bowel is located throughout the abdomen, characterized by large diameter and haustra.

7. B. Bile is secreted by the liver and is stored in the gallbladder. The liver also detoxifies substances from intestines, stores vitamins and performs hematopoiesis. Bile is transported from liver through left and right hepatic duct, which combines into the common hepatic duct. The common hepatic duct meets the cystic duct to form the common bile duct. On CT scan, the liver occupies most of the right side of the abdomen, extending to the midline. The gallbladder is inferior to liver, and darker in color than the liver on CT scans.

8. C. The pancreas produces insulin and digestive enzymes. This retroperitoneal structure has three parts: head (sits in "c" of duodenum at L1–L2), body (anterior to left kidney), and tail (medial to the spleen). The pancreatic duct meets common bile duct and enters the duodenum, and is commonly blocked by tumor. On CT scan, the pancreas sits midline in the abdominal cavity, anterior to the vertebral bodies. The head is near the duodenum, while the tail extends to the spleen. It has a unique, glandular texture.

9. C. There are approximately 16,500 new cases of esophageal cancer each year, and is more common in males than females. In addition to smoking, alcohol, and Barrett's esophagus, GERD, a poor diet and achalasia are also risk factors.

10. C. Tumors in the upper two-thirds of the esophagus are typically of squamous cell carcinoma histology, while tumors in the lower one-third are adenocarcinoma histology (increasing in incidence).

11. B. Spread of esophageal cancer may be direct (through the esophageal wall), lymphatic (skip metastasis are common), or distant routes (to liver and lungs). When designing radiation therapy treatment fields, the borders are drawn 5 cm superior and inferior due to lymph node skip metastasis.

12. B. Organs at risk when treating the esophagus with radiation therapy include the spinal cord, lung, heart, and stomach. Acute toxicities include esophagitis, myelosuppression, and fatigue, while late toxicities include stenosis and stricture of the esophagus.

13. D. Risk factors for stomach cancer include increased use of preservatives in food (especially in Japan), low socioeconomic status, *H. pylori*, tobacco, and family history.

14. A. Adenocarcinoma is the most common histology of stomach cancer, pancreatic cancer, and colorectal cancer.

15. D. Surgery is the primary treatment of stomach cancer. If the patient is inoperable, treatment is concomitant radiation therapy and chemotherapy. AP/PA fields or IMRT to the entire stomach, with a boost to the GTV is given to a total dose of 45–60 Gy. Treating with an empty stomach helps to decrease treatment volumes and avoid excess dose to the small bowel, heart, liver, kidneys, and spinal cord.

16. D. There are 148,000 new cases of colon cancer per year. Colon cancer is the third most common cancer overall in men and women, the most common GI malignancy, and the third most common cause of cancer deaths.

17. A. Risk factors for colorectal cancer include a diet high in fat and low in fiber, familial link (polyps), increased age, smoking, obesity, alcohol, and Crohn's disease.

18. C. Patients with colon cancer may present with polyps, change in stool, or hematochezia. Exams used to aid in the diagnosis of colorectal cancer include a digital rectal exam, fecal occult blood test, CT, MRI, and PET.
19. C. Duke's staging is used for colorectal cancer. Ann Arbor staging is used in Hodgkin's disease, FIGO staging in GYN malignancies, and Clarke's is used with skin cancers.
20. C. While the primary treatment for colorectal cancer is surgery (LAR or APR), rectal cancer is treated with preop or postop radiation therapy and chemotherapy (continuous infusion 5-FU). When treating rectal cancer with radiation therapy, patients are treated prone with PA and lateral fields, with wedges on lateral fields. The tumor and regional lymphatics are treated to a dose of 45 Gy, with a boost to the GTV to a total dose of 50–55 Gy.
21. A. Anal carcinomas are typically of squamous cell histology.
22. C. Rectal bleeding, pain, changes in bowel habits, and an anal mass are signs or symptoms of anal cancer.
23. A. Primary lymphatic drainage of anal cancer is to the superficial inguinal nodes, followed by the internal and external iliac lymph nodes. Anal cancer also spreads directly to the anal sphincter, rectum, vagina, and prostate and distantly to the liver and lungs.
24. D. Smoking, chronic pancreatitis, diabetes, and obesity are all risk factors for pancreatic cancer.
25. B. Pancreatic cancer often presents in advanced stage with jaundice (head of pancreas tumors), abdominal pain, anorexia, and weight loss.
26. B. CA 19–9 is used with pancreatic cancers. Other diagnostic exams include CT, endoscopic ultrasound, and ERCP.
27. A. Primary treatment of pancreatic cancer is the pancreatoduodectomy (Whipple surgery). If the tumor is unresectable, patients are treated with concurrent radiation therapy and chemotherapy (5-FU, gemcitabine). Four-field or IMRT radiation therapy is used to treat the tumor and regional lymphatics to a dose of 50.4–54 Gy. Gating or abdominal compression for treatment may be used to minimize movement of the tumor.
28. D. The prognosis of pancreatic cancer is very poor, with the 5-year overall survival less than 10 %.

Suggested Readings

Burdick MJ, Stephans KL. Gastrointestinal (non-esophageal radiotherapy). In: Videtic GMM, Vassil AD, editors. Handbook of treatment planning in radiation oncology. New York, NY: Demos Medical Publishing; 2011. p. 67–84.

Bussman-Yeakel L. Digestive system tumors. In: Washington CM, Leaver D, editors. Principles and practice of radiation therapy. 3rd ed. St. Louis, MO: Mosby Elsevier; 2010. p. 764–802.

Chao KSC. Colon and rectum. In: Chao KSC, Perez CA, Brady LW, editors. Radiation oncology management decisions. 3rd ed. Philadelphia, PA: Wolters Kluwer-Lippincott Williams and Wilkins; 2011. p. 443–54.

Hunter GK, Videtic GMM. Thoracic radiotherapy. In: Videtic GMM, Vassil AD, editors. Handbook of treatment planning in radiation oncology. New York, NY: Demos Medical Publishing; 2011. p. 85–100.

Madden M. Introduction of sectional anatomy. 2nd ed. Baltimore, MD: Wolters Kluwer-Lippincott Williams and Wilkins; 2008.

Shah AA, Chao KSC. Anal canal. In: Chao KSC, Perez CA, Brady LW, editors. Radiation oncology management decisions. 3rd ed. Philadelphia, PA: Wolters Kluwer-Lippincott Williams and Wilkins; 2011a. p. 455–68.

Shah AA, Chao KSC. Stomach. In: Chao KSC, Perez CA, Brady LW, editors. Radiation oncology management decisions. 3rd ed. Philadelphia, PA: Wolters Kluwer-Lippincott Williams and Wilkins; 2011b. p. 417–26.

Thibodeau G, Patton K. Anatomy and physiology. 5th ed. St. Louis, MO: Mosby- Elsevier; 2003.

Vann A, Dasher BG, Wiggers NH, Chesnut SK. Portal design in radiation therapy. 3rd ed. Augusta, GA: DWV Enterprises; 2013.

Chapter 16
Cancers of the Urinary System

Questions

1. The area in which the ureters and blood vessels enter and exit the kidneys is the:

    A. Nephron
    B. Hilum
    C. Minor calyx
    D. Renal sinus

2. The inferior border of the pyloric plane is:

    A. T12
    B. L1
    C. L2
    D. L3

3. The ureters enter the bladder through the _____ wall of the bladder.

    A. Superior
    B. Inferior
    C. Anterior
    D. Posterior

4. The bladder is posterior to the:

    A. Ilium
    B. Pubis bone
    C. Sacrum
    D. Obturator foramen

© Springer Science+Business Media New York 2016
A. Heath, *Radiation Therapy Study Guide*, DOI 10.1007/978-1-4939-3258-0_16

5. The lymphatics of the bladder include (choose all correct answers):

    A. Internal iliac nodes
    B. Para aortic nodes
    C. External iliac nodes
    D. Common iliac nodes
    E. Inguinal nodes

6. What is the average age of diagnosis for kidney cancer?

    A. 45–50 years old
    B. 50–55 years old
    C. 55–60 years old
    D. 60–65 years old

7. Which of the following is not a risk factor for kidney cancer?

    A. Obesity
    B. Smoking
    C. Leather tanning worker
    D. Alcohol use

8. What is a sign or symptom of kidney cancer?

    A. Hematuria
    B. Nocturia
    C. Urinary frequency
    D. Light stream

9. Which of the following is not a typical site for distant metastatic disease of the kidney?

    A. Brain
    B. Liver
    C. Lung
    D. Bone

10. Which is not a treatment modality used for kidney cancer?

    A. Interferon
    B. Interleukin
    C. Nephrectomy
    D. TURB

11. Which of the following is true regarding the epidemiology of bladder cancer?

    A. More common in females than males
    B. More common in males than females
    C. Fourth most common cancer in males
    D. More likely to occur in younger patients

12. The primary symptom of bladder cancer is:

    A. Painless hematuria
    B. Flank pain
    C. Palpable abdominal mass
    D. Urinary tract infection

13. The most common histology of bladder cancer is:

    A. Adenocarcinoma
    B. Squamous cell carcinoma
    C. Transitional cell carcinoma
    D. Clear cell carcinoma histology

14. The most common site within the bladder for cancer is:

    A. Base
    B. Trigone
    C. Apex
    D. Posterior wall

15. Which of the following is true regarding external beam radiation to the bladder? Choose all correct answers.

    A. Commonly used with chemotherapy
    B. Four-field beam arrangement
    C. Preferred modality of treatment
    D. Treat GTV to a total dose of 65–70 Gy
    E. Superior border is T10

16. In order to decrease toxicity to normal structures, you would instruct the patient to _____ during their boost treatment for bladder cancer.

    A. Fill their bladder
    B. Empty their bladder
    C. Fill their rectum
    D. Empty their rectum

Answers and Rationales

1. B. The hilum of the kidney is the depressed area where ureter and blood vessels enter and exit the kidney. The functional unit of the kidney is the nephron. The function of the kidney is to filter blood, remove waste, and form urine.

2. D. The kidneys are located lateral to the spine (between T12–L3) and are retroperitoneal. The right kidney is often lower than the left as a result of the liver pushing the right kidney inferior. On CT scan, the kidneys are located posterior in the body, lateral to the vertebral bodies, directly inferior to the liver on the right and spleen on the left.

3. D. The ureters connect the kidneys and bladder, entering the bladder through the posterior wall of the bladder at the trigone. The function of the ureters is to transport urine from the kidneys to the bladder.

4. B. The urinary bladder is a reservoir for urine; its size and shape changes with urine volume. Urine enters the bladder via the ureters and exits the bladder via urethra which forms the trigone of the bladder. On CT scan, the bladder is located between the pubis bone and rectum, filling the anterior portion of the pelvic cavity.

5. A, C, and D. Drainage of the bladder is the pelvic nodes: internal iliac nodes, external iliac nodes, and common iliac nodes.

6. B. There are 54,000 new cases of kidney cancer each year. The average age of diagnosis is 55–60 years old. Kidney cancer is more common in males than females.

7. D. Risk factors for kidney cancer include smoking, von Hippel-Lindau syndrome, obesity, and occupations such as leather tanners and petroleum workers.

8. A. In addition to hematuria, patients with kidney cancer may present with flank pain.

9. A. Kidney cancer may spread directly to the inferior vena cava, through the lymphatics or distantly to the lung, bone, and liver.

10. D. Primary treatment for kidney cancer is surgery (nephrectomy). Immunotherapy (interferon, interleukin) is also used. Primary treatment of bladder cancer is transurethral resection of bladder (TURB).

11. A. There are 69,000 new cases of bladder cancer each year. It is more common in males than females, and is the fourth most common cancer in men. Risk of bladder cancer increases with age, and is also linked to smoking, certain occupations (rubber and petroleum workers), chronic catheter use and schistosomiasis.

12. A. In addition to gross, painless hematuria, other signs and symptoms include urinary frequency and urgency, dysuria, and hydronephrosis.

13. C. Transitional cell is the most common histology of bladder cancer. In situ disease is common.

14. B. The trigone is the triangle in the inferior portion of the bladder, marked by the ureters and urethra

15. A, B, and D. Surgery is the primary treatment modality for bladder cancer, but combination chemotherapy (cisplatin) and radiation therapy may be used.

A four-field pelvis portal to include bladder and lymph nodes, followed by a boost to the bladder only. The pelvis is treated to 45–50 Gy, followed by boost to total dose of 65–70 Gy.

16. A. The pelvic field is treated with an empty bladder to decrease the treatment volume target, while the boost field is treated with a full bladder to decrease target volume and push small bowel out of the field. Acute side effects of treatment include cystitis, diarrhea, and fatigue, while late side effects include stricture, fibrosis, and obstruction.

Suggested Readings

Deutsch I. Bladder. In: Chao KSC, Perez CA, Brady LW, editors. Radiation oncology management decisions. 3rd ed. Philadelphia, PA: Wolters Kluwer-Lippincott Williams and Wilkins; 2011a. p. 483–94.

Deutsch I. Upper urinary tract. In: Chao KSC, Perez CA, Brady LW, editors. Radiation oncology management decisions. 3rd ed. Philadelphia, PA: Wolters Kluwer-Lippincott Williams and Wilkins; 2011b. p. 469–82.

Khan MK, Tendulkar RD, Stephans KL, Ciezki JP. Genitourinary radiotherapy. In: Videtic GMM, Vassil AD, editors. Handbook of treatment planning in radiation oncology. New York, NY: Demos Medical Publishing; 2011. p. 117–42.

Kuban DA, Trad ML. Male reproductive and genitourinary tumors. In: Washington CM, Leaver D, editors. Principles and practice of radiation therapy. 3rd ed. St. Louis, MO: Mosby Elsevier; 2010. p. 823–65.

Madden M. Introduction of sectional anatomy. 2nd ed. Baltimore, MD: Wolters Kluwer-Lippincott Williams and Wilkins; 2008.

Thibodeau G, Patton K. Anatomy and physiology. 5th ed. St. Louis, MO: Mosby-Elsevier; 2003.

Vann A, Dasher BG, Wiggers NH, Chesnut SK. Portal design in radiation therapy. 3rd ed. Augusta, GA: DWV Enterprises; 2013.

Chapter 17
Cancers of the Male Reproductive System

Questions

1. What organ of the male reproductive system produces sperm?

   A. Testes
   B. Epididymis
   C. Seminal vesicles
   D. Prostate

2. The seminal vesicles are located _____ to the prostate.

   A. Anterior
   B. Posterior
   C. Superior
   D. Inferior

3. The prostate is _____ to the rectum and _____ to the bladder.

   A. Anterior, posterior
   B. Anterior, inferior
   C. Superior, posterior
   D. Superior, inferior

4. Primary lymphatic drainage of the prostate is:

   A. Para-aortic nodes
   B. Inguinal nodes
   C. Common iliac nodes
   D. Obturator nodes

© Springer Science+Business Media New York 2016
A. Heath, *Radiation Therapy Study Guide*, DOI 10.1007/978-1-4939-3258-0_17

5. Primary lymphatic drainage of the testes is:

   A. Para-aortic nodes
   B. Inguinal nodes
   C. Common iliac nodes
   D. Obturator nodes

6. _____ is a risk factor for testicular cancer.

   A. Increased age
   B. Hispanic ethnicity
   C. Cryptorchidism
   D. Trauma to the testicles

7. A tumor marker used to aid in the diagnosis of testicular cancer is:

   A. CA 19-9
   B. PSA
   C. AFP
   D. HER2/neu

8. Primary treatment of testicular cancer is:

   A. Surgery
   B. Chemotherapy
   C. Observation
   D. Radiation therapy

9. The superior border for treatment fields when treating testicular cancer with external beam radiation therapy is:

   A. T8
   B. T10
   C. T12
   D. L2

10. What is not true regarding radiation therapy treatment for testicular cancer?

    A. The orchiectomy scar must be included in the treatment field
    B. Late toxicity includes infertility
    C. Nausea and vomiting are a common acute side effect
    D. Lower dose per fraction is used to decrease acute toxicities

11. The most prevalent cancer in males is:

    A. Prostate cancer
    B. Testicular cancer
    C. Bladder cancer
    D. Kidney cancer

12. What is not a primary diagnostic test for prostate cancer?

    A. Digital rectal exam (DRE)
    B. Prostate-specific antigen (PSA)
    C. PET
    D. Transrectal biopsy

13. What is the most common histology of prostate cancer?

    A. Transitional cell carcinoma
    B. Clear-cell carcinoma
    C. Adenocarcinoma
    D. Squamous cell carcinoma

14. Distantly, prostate cancer spreads to the:

    A. Liver
    B. Bone
    C. Lungs
    D. Brain

15. Which is not an acceptable treatment option for early-staged prostate cancer?

    A. Hypofractionated radiation therapy
    B. Prostatectomy
    C. Brachytherapy
    D. Hockeystick radiation therapy

16. When treating prostate cancer using conventional fractionation to the prostate, the typical total dose should be:

    A. 78 Gy
    B. 50.4 Gy
    C. 66 Gy
    D. 72 Gy

17. Which of the following are organs at risk when treating prostate cancer with IMRT? Choose all correct answers.

    A. Femoral heads
    B. Small bowel
    C. Rectum
    D. Bladder

18. Which radioactive isotope may be used when treating the prostate with brachytherapy?

    A. Pd 103
    B. Sm 93
    C. I 121
    D. Au 43

19. Prostate patients experiencing diarrhea may be advised to follow a _____ diet.

    A. High fiber
    B. Low residue
    C. High fat
    D. Gluten free

Answers and Rationales

1. A. The testes produce sperm, which fertilize female ova to produce offspring. The epididymis serves as a place for sperm maturation and pathway for sperm. The seminal vesicles secrete alkaline fluid, which is added to seminal fluid. The prostate also adds sections to seminal fluid.

2. C. The seminal vesicles are glands located superior to the prostate, between the bladder and rectum. On CT scan, the seminal vesicles are located on slices superior to the prostate and seen posterior to the bladder and anterior to the rectum.

3. B. The prostate is glandular tissue anterior the rectum and inferior to bladder, encompassing the urethra. It lies posterior to pubis symphysis. On CT scan, the soft tissue structure is located between the base of the bladder and rectum. Is difficult to identify in slices where the bladder is not present; urethral contrast will aid in identification.

4. D. Primary lymphatic drainage of the prostate is the obturator lymph nodes. Next, lymph travels through hypogastric, internal iliac, external iliac, and common iliac nodes.

5. A. Para-aortic lymph nodes are the primary lymphatic drainage of the testes. Ipsilateral pelvic lymph nodes may also be involved.

6. C. History of cryptorchidism (undescended testicle) is a risk factor of testicular cancer. Testicular cancer is more common in Caucasians, and younger adult males. Testicular cancer often presents as a painless lump in the testicle, found on self-exam.

7. C. In addition to ultrasound and CT, alpha fetoprotein (AFP) is used to diagnose testicular cancer.

8. A. Surgery is the primary treatment of testicular cancer, as all patients undergo orchiectomy. Seminoma patients may have postoperative radiation therapy to regional lymphatics and nonseminoma patients may have postoperative chemo-therapy (cisplatin).

9. B. AP/PA para-aortic fields or hockey stick fields (treats para aortic nodes and ipsilateral pelvic nodes) are used for testicular cancer, with the patient supine and frog-legged. The borders are as follows:

   - Superior: T10
   - Inferior: L4–L5 (para-aortic); Bottom ischial tuberosity (hockeystick)
   - Centered midline, 9–10 cm wide, hockeystick field angled at level of L4

10. A. The orchiectomy scar does not need to be included in the treatment field. Scrotal shields are used to block scatter dose to testes. A total dose of 25–30 Gy is prescribed, with a lower dose per fraction to decrease acute toxicities. Acute toxicities include nausea and vomiting (patient needs antiemetic), decreased sperm count, and myelosuppression. Late toxicity is infertility, and patients should be advised to undergo sperm banking prior to treatment.

11. A. There are 200,000 new cases of prostate cancer each year. Prostate cancer is the most prevalent cancer in men and the second cause of cancer deaths in men.

Incidence is higher in African-American men than Caucasian men. In addition, incidence increases with age and family history.

12. C. In addition to DRE, PSA, and transrectal biopsies, pelvic CT and bone scans are also used in the diagnosis of prostate cancer.

13. C. The histology of prostate cancer is adenocarcinoma. Gleason score indicates grade.

14. B. Prostate cancer spreads directly to the seminal vesicles, bladder, and rectum. Lymphatic drainage is to the obturator nodes, hypogastric nodes, external iliac nodes, and common iliac nodes. Distantly, prostate cancer spreads to the bone (lytic lesions).

15. D. Patients have many options for primary treatment. Options include surgery (radical prostatectomy), radiation therapy (external beam or brachytherapy) or observation. Hormonal treatment (androgen deprivation drugs) may be added, such as Lupron, Casodex, and Megace.

16. A. External beam treatment is often delivered via IMRT, with six to seven fields to prostate and seminal vesicles to 78 Gy. If lymph node coverage is required, patients are treated with a four field pelvis fields to an initial dose of 45 Gy, followed by boost to the prostate to 78 Gy.

17. A, C, and D. Organs at risk when treating the prostate only include the rectum, bladder, and femoral heads. The small bowel is at risk when treating the lymph nodes and pelvis. Patients may be treated prone in order to move the small bowel out of the field for these patients.

18. A. Common isotopes used for brachytherapy include I-125 and Pd-103.

19. B. Prostate cancer patients receiving radiation to the pelvis should follow a low-residue diet to minimize diarrhea.

Suggested Readings

Deutsch I. Prostate. In: Chao KSC, Perez CA, Brady LW, editors. Radiation oncology management decisions. 3rd ed. Philadelphia, PA: Wolters Kluwer-Lippincott Williams and Wilkins; 2011a. p. 495–521.

Deutsch I. Testis. In: Chao KSC, Perez CA, Brady LW, editors. Radiation oncology management decisions. 3rd ed. Philadelphia, PA: Wolters Kluwer-Lippincott Williams and Wilkins; 2011b. p. 523–37.

Khan MK, Tendulkar RD, Stephans KL, Ciezki JP. Genitourinary radiotherapy. In: Videtic GMM, Vassil AD, editors. Handbook of treatment planning in radiation oncology. New York: Demos Medical Publishing; 2011. p. 117–42.

Kuban DA, Trad ML. Male reproductive and genitourinary tumors. In: Washington CM, Leaver D, editors. Principles and practice of radiation therapy. 3rd ed. St. Louis, MO: Mosby Elsevier; 2010. p. 823–65.

Madden M. Introduction of sectional anatomy. 2nd ed. Baltimore, MD: Wolters Kluwer-Lippincott Williams and Wilkins; 2008.

Thibodeau G, Patton K. Anatomy and physiology. 5th ed. St. Louis, MO: Mosby-Elsevier; 2003.

Vann A, Dasher BG, Wiggers NH, Chesnut SK. Portal design in radiation therapy. 3rd ed. Augusta, GA: DWV Enterprises; 2013.

Chapter 18
Cancers of the Female Reproductive System

Questions

1. The essential organ(s) of the female reproductive system is the:

    A. Fallopian tubes
    B. Ovary
    C. Uterus
    D. Vagina

2. The uterus is located posterior to the:

    A. Obturator foramen
    B. Rectum
    C. Abdominal aorta
    D. Bladder

3. This layer of the uterus is shed during menstruation:

    A. Endometrium
    B. Myometrium
    C. Parietal peritoneum
    D. All are shed during menstruation

4. The most inferior portion of the uterus is the:

    A. Cervix
    B. Fundus
    C. Body
    D. Vagina

© Springer Science+Business Media New York 2016
A. Heath, *Radiation Therapy Study Guide*, DOI 10.1007/978-1-4939-3258-0_18

5. The structure posterior to the vagina is the:

    A. Bladder
    B. Rectum
    C. Labia major
    D. Labia minor

6. The primary lymphatic drainage of the vulva are the:

    A. Para-aortic nodes
    B. Inguinal nodes
    C. Obturator nodes
    D. External iliac nodes

7. What female hormone promotes initial duct development in the breasts?

    A. Estrogen
    B. Prolactin
    C. Progesterone
    D. Oxytocin

8. Level 2 axillary nodes are located:

    A. Superior to the pectoralis muscle
    B. Lateral to the sternum
    C. Under the pectoralis muscle
    D. Under and lateral to the pectoralis muscle

9. Which gynecological cancer causes the most deaths per year?

    A. Endometrial
    B. Vaginal
    C. Ovarian
    D. Vulvar

10. What of the following is a risk factor for cervical cancer?

    A. Human papilloma virus
    B. BRCA gene
    C. Diethylstebesterol (DES) use by mother when in utero
    D. Early menarche

11. The most common gynecological cancer is cancer of the:

    A. Uterus
    B. Cervix
    C. Ovary
    D. Vulva

12. Which gynecological cancer presents with ascites?

   A. Uterus
   B. Cervix
   C. Ovary
   D. Vulva

13. Papanicolaou smears are used to detect cancer of the:

   A. Uterus
   B. Cervix
   C. Ovary
   D. Vagina

14. What tumor marker can be used for ovarian cancer?

   A. PSA
   B. CA-125
   C. CEA
   D. CA 19-9

15. What is the most common histology of endometrial cancer?

   A. Clear cell
   B. Squamous cell carcinoma
   C. Adenocarcinoma
   D. Small-cell carcinoma

16. Which of the following is not true regarding treatment for ovarian cancer?

   A. I-131 washings of the peritoneal cavity are used
   B. The superior border of whole abdomen radiation therapy is higher on the right side
   C. Partial kidney and liver blocks are used in whole abdomen treatment
   D. Cisplatin and cyclophosphamide is used postoperatively

17. Which of the following is not a sign or symptom of cervical cancer?

   A. Postcoital bleeding
   B. Painful intercourse
   C. Vaginal discharge
   D. Pruritis

18. Primary lymphatic drainage of the cervix are the:

   A. Obturator nodes
   B. Inguinal nodes
   C. Para-aortic nodes
   D. Nodal spread is not common

19. What is not a treatment option for cervical cancer?

    A. Tandem and ovoid brachytherapy
    B. TAHBSO
    C. External radiation therapy to the pelvis
    D. Whole-abdomen radiation therapy

20. What is the most common sign or symptom of endometrial cancer?

    A. Abnormal vaginal bleeding
    B. Abnormal vaginal discharge
    C. Pelvic pain
    D. Painful intercourse

21. When treating the pelvis for gynecological cancer, what is not an organ at risk?

    A. Bladder
    B. Small bowel
    C. Liver
    D. Rectum

22. Late toxicities of external beam radiation therapy treatment to the pelvis include all of the following except:

    A. Diarrhea
    B. Fibrosis
    C. Stenosis
    D. Enteritis

23. What is common organ for distant spread of endometrial cancer?

    A. Cervix
    B. External iliac nodes
    C. Lung
    D. Bladder

24. Vaginal cancer is typically _____ histology.

    A. Clear cell
    B. Squamous cell
    C. Adenocarcinoma
    D. Epithelial carcinoma

25. Which of the following techniques would not be used to treat cervical cancer?

    A. Concomitant chemoradiotherapy
    B. Interstitial brachytherapy
    C. Whole-abdomen radiation therapy
    D. Whole-pelvis radiation therapy

26. Vulvar cancers primarily spread to the

    A. Superficial inguinal nodes
    B. Para-aortic nodes
    C. Common iliac nodes
    D. Femoral nodes

27. The most common cancer in women is:

    A. Endometrial cancer
    B. Cervical cancer
    C. Breast cancer
    D. Vulvar cancer

28. Which of the following is true regarding the risk of developing breast cancer?

    A. Risk is higher in younger patients
    B. Risk is lower in patients with late menopause
    C. Family history does not have an impact
    D. Risk is lower in patients with late menarche

29. Which of the following is not a common sign or symptom of breast cancer?

    A. Painless, palpable mass
    B. Enlarged supraclavicular lymph node
    C. Skin changes (peau d'orange)
    D. Nipple changes, retraction, or discharge

30. The most common histology of breast cancer is:

    A. Infiltrating ductal carcinoma
    B. Ductal carcinoma in situ
    C. Lobular carcinoma
    D. Inflammatory carcinoma

31. Which is not a test commonly used to diagnose breast cancer?

    A. Self-breast exam
    B. Mammogram
    C. CT of the chest and abdomen
    D. Ultr asound

32. What is not a common distant metastatic site for breast cancer spread?

    A. Lung
    B. Bone
    C. Brain
    D. Muscle

33. Which of the following is a hormonal treatment used for the treatment of breast cancer?

    A. Tamoxifen
    B. Lupron
    C. Casodex
    D. Coumadin

34. A posterior-axillary-boost (PAB) field is used to increase the dose to what lymph node group?

    A. Level 1 axillary nodes
    B. Level 2 axillary nodes
    C. Level 3 axillary nodes
    D. Supraclavicular nodes

35. Which of the following is not true regarding radiation therapy for breast cancer?

    A. Internal mammary nodes are typically included in deep tangent fields
    B. Lumpectomy boosts are only treated with electrons
    C. Patients may be supine, on a slant board or prone
    D. Patients with left-sided disease may be treated with breath holds

36. The inferior border of a tangent breast field is:

    A. Fifth intercostal space
    B. 1.5 cm inferior to breast tissue
    C. First intercostal space
    D. Midaxillary line

37. What is not true regarding treatment of supraclavicular fields when treating a patient with breast cancer?

    A. Gantry is angled 10–15° towards the affected side
    B. Inferior border is half-beam blocked
    C. Medial border is 1 cm past midline
    D. Lateral border bisects the humeral head

38. Which of the following does not accurately describe the dose and fractionation when treating breast cancer?

    A. 45–60 Gy is delivered to the breast and nodal tissue
    B. If a boost is used, the tumor volume is treated to a total dose to 60–66 Gy
    C. Dose may be hyperfractionated
    D. Partial breast radiation may be treated via brachytherapy

39. Following radiation therapy to the breast, what is a late toxicity to the skin?

    A. Telangectasia
    B. Erythema
    C. Inflammation
    D. Moist desquamation

40. What is true regarding the prognosis of breast cancer?

    A. Overall survival is 89 %

    B. Patients with negative hormone status have a better prognosis

    C. Lymph node status has no effect on disease-free survival rates

    D. Increased tumor size at diagnosis improves prognosis

41. Which of the following are risk factors for breast cancer? Choose all that apply.

    A. Increased age

    B. Late menopause

    C. Von Hippel Lindau disease

    D. Family history

    E. Epstein-Barr virus

42. Brachytherapy is not typically used to treat:

    A. Early-stage ovarian cancer

    B. Breast cancer

    C. Cervical cancer

    D. Endometrial cancer

Answers and Rationales

1. B. The ovaries are the essential organ of the reproductive system, and produce ova which are released during ovulation.
2. D. The pear-shaped uterus is located posterior to the bladder and anterior to the rectum.
3. A. The uterus serves as reproductive tract, site of fertilization, and site of implantation if fertilization occurs. If fertilization does not occur, endometrial layer is shed during menstruation.
4. A. The part of the uterus include the fundus (upper portion), body (middle portion) and cervix (inferior portion). The internal os is the cervical opening into body of uterus and the external os is the vaginal opening to the cervix. Primary blood supply of the uterus is from the uterine artery, a branch of the internal iliac arteries. It is held in place by the broad ligaments, along with others.
5. B. The vagina is located anterior to the rectum, posterior to the bladder, and between labia major and minor. The vaginal fornix is the area at which the vagina meets the cervix. The vagina is difficult to visualize on CT scan without radiopaque markers placed, which helps to identify the vaginal wall.
6. B. The vulva and other external genitalia drain to the inguinal lymph nodes, located in the groin. Other organs of the female reproductive system follow the blood supply of the pelvis, draining to the internal and external iliac chain, then the common iliac nodes, and up to the para-aortic nodes.
7. A. Estrogen promotes initial duct development, while progesterone completes the development. Prolactin and oxytocin, which is released after birth, stimulates milk production and ejection.
8. C. Primary lymphatics of the breast include the axillary lymphatics, levels 1–3. Level 1 are located under and lateral to pectoralis minor muscle, level 2 are located under pectoralis muscle, and level 3 are located superior to pectoralis muscle, near coracoid process of scapula. Internal mammary nodes may also be involved, which are very superficial, located lateral to the sternum.
9. C. Ovarian cancer is the second most common gynecological cancer, but causes the most gynecological cancer deaths per year.
10. A. HPV status, high number of sexual partners and low socioeconomic status are all risk factors for cervical cancer. Few or late pregnancies, late menopause, BRCA+, and a diet high in fat are risk factors for ovarian cancer. Risk for clear cell vaginal cancer is increased with DES use by mother in utero. Early menarche is linked to endometrial cancer.
11. A. There are approximately 39,000 new cases of cancer of the uterus each year. Vulvar and vaginal cancer are the most uncommon.
12. C. There are no early warning signs for ovarian cancer, and patients often present at a late stage with abdominal pain, ascites, and abdominal distension.
13. B. Other tests used to detect and diagnose cervical cancer include pelvic exams, colposcopy and biopsy, and CT and MRI of the pelvis.
14. B. CA-125 is the tumor marker used to diagnose and detect ovarian cancer.

15. C. Adenocarcinoma is the most common histology of endometrial cancer. Cancers of the cervix, vagina, and vulva are typically of squamous cell histology, while ovarian cancers are germ cell in nature.

16. A. Treatment of ovarian cancer may include surgery and postop chemotherapy (cisplatin and cyclophosphamide), P32 washings of peritoneal cavity, and whole-abdomen radiation therapy (though rarely used). Whole abdomen treatment is given to a total dose of 25–28 Gy via AP/PA fields, with the following borders used:

   - Superior: 2 cm superior to diaphragm (higher on right side due to liver)
   - Inferior: Bottom obturator foramen
   - Lateral: Include peritoneum without flashing skin
   - Partial kidney and liver blocks may be used

17. D. Cervical cancers can also be asymptomatic and found through Papanicolaou smear. Pruritis is common in patients with vulvar cancer.

18. A. Primary lymphatic drainage of cervical cancer is through the obturator and iliac nodes. Cervical cancer also spreads directly to adjacent tissue, parametrium, bladder, and rectum. Distantly, cervical cancer spreads to the lungs, para-aortic nodes, bones, and liver.

19. D. Treatment for cervical cancer may include TAHBSO + Vaginal Cuff Brachytherapy or T&O Brachytherapy alone for Stage 1 disease. Stage 2–4 disease is often treated with pelvic radiation + chemotherapy (cisplatin) with brachytherapy boost.

20. A. Abnormal vaginal bleeding is the most common presentation of endometrial cancer, though abnormal vaginal discharge and pelvic pain may also be experienced.

21. C. When treating a patient with four field pelvis fields, the organs at risk include the bladder, rectum, small bowel, femoral heads, ovaries, kidneys. Patients may be treated prone in a bellyboard to decrease small bowel dose. In addition a midline block may be added to the fields during brachytherapy boost.

22. A. Acute toxicities when treating the pelvis for gynecological cancers include diarrhea, skin changes, fatigue, urinary symptoms, and myelosuppression. Late toxicities include fibrosis, stenosis, fistulas, and enteritis.

23. C. Direct spread of endometrial cancer includes extension through parametrium and to the cervix, bladder, vagina, and rectum. Lymphatic spread is through the internal and external iliac nodes and distant spread is to the lung and liver.

24. B. Vaginal cancers are typically squamous cell histology.

25. C. Whole-abdomen radiation therapy is a treatment for ovarian cancer, not cervical cancer.

26. A. Primary lymphatic drainage of the vulva is the superficial inguinal nodes.

27. C. Breast cancer is the most common cancer in women, with 182,000 new cases per year. The most common location is left breast, upper outer quadrant.

28. D. Risk factors for breast cancer include: age (incidence increases with increasing age), family history (BRCA1 and BRCA2 genes), early menarche and late menopause (estrogen and progesterone link), and previous radiation to the chest.

29. B. In addition, many breast cancers are often asymptomatic, and found on mammogram.
30. A. Infiltrating ductal carcinoma is the most common histology of breast cancer.
31. C. Self-breast exams and mammograms are commonly used. MRI may be used for dense breasts. Ultrasound is helpful to distinguish between a cyst and mass in the breast. In addition fine needle aspiration or core biopsy may be used to obtain tissue for pathology. ER/PR status and Her2neu is also assessed.
32. D. Breast cancer can spread distantly to the brain, lung and bone.
33. A. In addition to surgery, chemotherapy and radiation therapy, hormonal therapy may be used in the treatment of breast cancer. Tamoxifen and Herceptin are two common hormonal therapies used.
34. C. Radiation therapy fields include medial and lateral tangents, with or without supraclavicular and posterior axillary boost (PAB) fields, as well as lumpectomy boost. The supraclavicular field is added when patient has four or more positive lymphnodes or extracapsular extension. A PAB field is used when level 3 axillary nodes are not getting adequate dose, or when patient has extensive nodal disease.
35. B. While internal mammary nodes are typically included in deep tangent fields, they may also be treated with a separate electron field. Lumpectomy boosts were traditionally treated with electrons, but now may be treated with photons due to 3D treatment planning. In addition to external beam radiation therapy, interstitial brachytherapy, or accelerated partial breast irradiation (APBI) are commonly used with early-stage disease.
36. B. Tangent field borders are as follows:

    Superior: First intercostal space
    Inferior: 1.5 cm below breast tissue (wire may be used at simulation to identify location of breast tissue on imaging)
    Medial: Midline
    Lateral: Midaxillary line

37. A. With supraclavicular fields, the gantry is angled 10–15° away from affected side to avoid esophagus and spinal cord. Borders are as follows:

    Superior: Do not flash skin
    Inferior: Match superior border of tangents, half-beam block to match divergence
    Medial: 1 cm past midline
    Lateral: Bisect humeral head

38. C. Breast and nodal volume is treated to a dose of 45–60 Gy, and may not be boosted to a total dose of 60–66 Gy. The dose may be hypofractionated. Brachytherapy is used in early-stage disease.
39. A. Organs at risk when designing radiation therapy fields for breast cancer include the lung, heart, humeral head, esophagus, spinal cord, brachial plexus, and contralateral breast. Acute toxicities are skin reactions, fatigue, and

esophagitis, while late toxicities include telangectasia, pneumonitis, heart disease, and brachialplexopathy.

40. A. The overall prognosis of breast cancer is approximately 89 %. Prognostic factors include: lymph node status, histology, grade, tumor size, and hormone status (negative status has worse prognosis).

41. A, B, and D. Risk factors for breast cancer include: increased age, increased estrogen exposure (nulliparity, early menarche, late menopause), and family history (linked to BRCA1 and BRCA2 gene).

42. A. Brachytherapy is used for the treatment of breast, cervical, and endometrial cancer.

Suggested Readings

Guo S, Juliano JJ. Gynecologic radiotherapy. In: Videtic GMM, Vassil AD, editors. Handbook of treatment planning in radiation oncology. New York: Demos Medical Publishing; 2011. p. 143–56.

Madden M. Introduction of sectional anatomy. 2nd ed. Baltimore, MD: Wolters Kluwer-Lippincott Williams and Wilkins; 2008.

Patel P, Wernicke AG. Uterine cervix. In: Chao KSC, Perez CA, Brady LW, editors. Radiation oncology management decisions. 3rd ed. Philadelphia, PA: Wolters Kluwer-Lippincott Williams and Wilkins; 2011a. p. 555–78.

Patel P, Wernicke AG. Endometrium. In: Chao KSC, Perez CA, Brady LW, editors. Radiation oncology management decisions. 3rd ed. Philadelphia, PA: Wolters Kluwer-Lippincott Williams and Wilkins; 2011b. p. 579–90.

Thibodeau G, Patton K. Anatomy and physiology. 5th ed. St. Louis, MO: Mosby-Elsevier; 2003.

Uschold GM, Anderson JE. Gynecological tumors. In: Washington CM, Leaver D, editors. Principles and practice of radiation therapy. 3rd ed. St. Louis, MO: Mosby Elsevier; 2010. p. 803–22.

Uschold GM, Zhang H. Breast cancer. In: Washington CM, Leaver D, editors. Principles and practice of radiation therapy. 3rd ed. St. Louis, MO: Mosby Elsevier; 2010. p. 866–94.

Vann A, Dasher BG, Wiggers NH, Chesnut SK. Portal design in radiation therapy. 3rd ed. Augusta, GA: DWV Enterprises; 2013.

Vassil AD, Tendulkar RD. Breast radiotherapy. In: Videtic GMM, Vassil AD, editors. Handbook of treatment planning in radiation oncology. New York: Demos Medical Publishing; 2011. p. 67–84.

Wernicke AG. Ovary and fallopian tube. In: Chao KSC, Perez CA, Brady LW, editors. Radiation oncology management decisions. 3rd ed. Philadelphia, PA: Wolters Kluwer-Lippincott Williams and Wilkins; 2011a. p. 591–608.

Wernicke AG. Vagina. In: Chao KSC, Perez CA, Brady LW, editors. Radiation oncology management decisions. 3rd ed. Philadelphia, PA: Wolters Kluwer-Lippincott Williams and Wilkins; 2011b. p. 609–22.

Wernicke AG. Vulva. In: Chao KSC, Perez CA, Brady LW, editors. Radiation oncology management decisions. 3rd ed. Philadelphia, PA: Wolters Kluwer-Lippincott Williams and Wilkins; 2011c. p. 623–38.

Chapter 19
Oncology Review

Questions

1. Which of the following is true regarding leukemia?

    A. AML is the primary subtype of leukemia in children
    B. Chronic leukemia is more prevalent that acute leukemia
    C. Exposure to ionizing radiation is a risk factor for developing leukemia
    D. ALL is common in patients over the age of 40

2. Leukemia often presents with thrombocytopenia, expressed in patients by (choose all correct answers):

    A. Petichae
    B. Alopecia
    C. Epitaxis
    D. Edema

3. Which of the following is NOT a primary test used when diagnosing leukemia?

    A. Complete blood count
    B. Bone marrow biopsy
    C. Immunophenotyping histological tests
    D. MRI

4. CML stands for:

    A. Chronic myelogenous leukemia
    B. Consistent myelogenous leukemia
    C. Chronic myeloid leukemia
    D. Consistent myelogenous leukemia

5. Which is true regarding the use of chemotherapy for treatment of leukemia? Choose all correct answers.

   A. It is not useful, as leukemia is a localized disease
   B. It is administered via induction, consolidation, and maintenance phases
   C. It is the primary treatment modality for leukemia
   D. It is only used for palliative cases

6. Autologous bone marrow transplants are when the bone marrow donor is:

   A. The patient
   B. An identical twin
   C. A blood relative
   D. An unrelated donor

7. Which is true regarding total body irradiation prior to a bone marrow transplant? Choose all correct answers.

   A. Patients are treated twice per day
   B. Patients are treated at an extended distance
   C. The head, lungs, and feet are blocked
   D. Patients are treated to a total dose of 18 Gy
   E. Patients are often in neutropenic precautions

8. When treating CNS disease in ALL patients using a whole brain field, the inferior border is typically at:

   A. C1
   B. C2
   C. EAM
   D. Occipital condyles

9. The incidence of Hodgkin's disease:

   A. Is most common amongst 25–30-year-olds
   B. Has a peak in incidence in elderly patients
   C. Is classified as bimodal age distribution
   D. All of the above

10. _____ virus is linked to the development of Hodgkin's disease.

   A. Human papilloma
   B. Epstein-Barr
   C. Human immunodeficiency
   D. Human herpes virus 8

11. Which of the following is not a B symptom?

   A. Night sweats
   B. Fever
   C. Petechiae
   D. Weight loss

12. Which subtype of Hodgkin's disease is the most common?

   A. Mixed cellularity
   B. Nodular sclerosing
   C. Lymphocytic predominant
   D. Lymphocytic depleted

13. Pathologically, the presence of _____ indicates a Hodgkin's disease diagnosis.

   A. P-53 mutation
   B. Reed-Sternberg cells
   C. NK cells
   D. Granular lymphocytes

14. The _____ staging system is commonly used to describe the extent of Hodgkin's disease.

   A. Ann Arbor
   B. Duke's
   C. FIGO
   D. Clarke's

15. Unlike non-Hodgkin's lymphoma, Hodgkin's disease spreads in a _____ manner.

   A. Arbitrary
   B. Contiguous
   C. Random
   D. Indiscriminate

16. Treatment for Hodgkin's disease may include all of the following except:

   A. MOPP chemotherapy
   B. Interleukin
   C. Radiation therapy to involved nodes
   D. AVBD chemotherapy

17. The inferior border of a mantle field is placed around:

   A. T4
   B. T7
   C. T10
   D. L1

18. Which of the following may be long term toxicities of mantle irradiation? Choose all correct answers.

   A. Secondary malignancies
   B. Myelosuppression
   C. Dysphagia
   D. Hypothyroidism

19. Which of the following is not true regarding inverted Y fields?

    A. The inferior border is a the L4/L5 interspace
    B. Shielding or transposition of the reproductive organs is offered to patients
    C. Dose may fall between 20 and 36 Gy, depending on bulkiness of disease
    D. Field width is 8–10 cm

20. Organs at risk identified when treating with inverted Y fields include (choose all correct answers):

    A. Ovaries
    B. Liver
    C. Kidney
    D. Spleen
    E. Large intestine

21. Which of the following is not true regarding non-Hodgkin's lymphoma?

    A. Average age at diagnosis is 65 years of age
    B. Development has been linked to occupational and environmental exposures
    C. Non-Hodgkin's lymphoma is less common in the USA than Hodgkin's disease
    D. Exposure to ionizing radiation is a risk factor

22. Which of the following is not a common site for non-Hodgkin's lymphoma?

    A. CNS
    B. GI organs
    C. Waldeyer's ring
    D. Ovaries

23. Which chemotherapy agents are commonly used for the treatment of non-Hodgkin's lymphoma?

    A. CHOP
    B. Cisplatin
    C. Adriamyacin
    D. Bleomyacin

24. Which of the following is true regarding thyroid cancer?

    A. It is more common in males
    B. It can be caused by radiation exposure
    C. Accounts for 12 % of all cancers
    D. Is the least prevalent endocrine tumor

25. All of the following are used to diagnose thyroid tumors, except:

    A. PET
    B. Ultrasound
    C. Thyroid function labwork
    D. Fine-needle aspiration

26. Which histology is the most aggressive thyroid cancer?

    A. Anaplastic
    B. Papillary
    C. Follicular
    D. Medullary

27. Which histology of thyroid cancer is most likely to spread distantly to the bone and lung?

    A. Anaplastic
    B. Papillary
    C. Follicular
    D. Medullary

28. What isotope is used to treat thyroid cancer?

    A. I-125
    B. Pd-103
    C. I-131
    D. Sr-90

29. Which of the following is not true regarding pituitary cancer?

    A. Patients often present with hormonal changes
    B. Tumors can cause headaches and visual changes
    C. MRI is the primary diagnostic tool
    D. Tumors are usually malignant

30. What treatment technique is not commonly used for pituitary tumors?

    A. Arc radiation therapy treatment, with a total dose of 45–50.4 Gy
    B. IMRT treatment, with a total dose of 20–25 Gy
    C. SRS, with a total dose of 15–25 Gy
    D. Transphenoidal hypophysectomy

31. If treating a pituitary tumor with external beam radiation, what structures are identified as organs at risk? Choose all correct answers.

    A. Optic nerve
    B. Spinal cord
    C. Lens of the eye
    D. Cerebrum
    E. Mandible

32. Approximately _____ cases of skin cancer are diagnosed each year.

    A. 10,000
    B. 100,000
    C. 1,000,000
    D. >1,000,000

33. Which of the following are risk factors for developing skin cancers (choose all correct answers):

    A. Sun exposure
    B. Fair complexion
    C. Alcohol consumption
    D. Previous skin cancer

34. Which of the following is not a sign or symptom of skin cancer?

    A. Skin lesion with asymmetry
    B. Sore that does not heal
    C. Skin lesion that stays the same size over time
    D. Skin lesion with irregular pigmentation

35. Which histology of skin cancer would most likely warrant a complete work-up following initial diagnosis via a biopsy?

    A. Melanoma
    B. Squamous cell carcinoma
    C. Basal cell carcinoma
    D. All of the above would need a complete work-up.

36. Which histology of skin cancers is most common?

    A. Melanoma
    B. Squamous cell carcinoma
    C. Basal cell carcinoma
    D. Merkel cell carcinoma

37. Immunotherapy has been used to treat which histology of skin cancer?

    A. Melanoma
    B. Squamous cell carcinoma
    C. Basal cell carcinoma
    D. Merkel cell carcinoma

38. _____ is a type of surgery in which layer by layer of skin is removed until no cancer is present.

    A. Moh's surgery
    B. Whipple technique
    C. Incisional biopsy
    D. Halstead surgical procedure

39. Which of the following does not accurately describe the radiation therapy treatment for a basal cell carcinoma of the skin?

    A. May be treated with electrons
    B. 3–4 cm margin is added to the lesion when designing the treatment fields
    C. Total dose of 50–60 Gy is used
    D. Lead blocks may be used to block backscatter

40. Which skin change is a late toxicity?

    A. Erythema
    B. Fibrosis
    C. Moist desquamation
    D. Dry desquamation

41. What statements accurately describe the epidemiology and etiology of primary bone tumors? Choose all correct answers.

    A. Common malignancy with annual incidence of 24,000 cases per year
    B. More common in males than females
    C. Common in patients over 50 years old
    D. Has a genetic link
    E. Can be attributed to numerous growth spurts during childhood

42. The most common indication of a primary bone tumor is:

    A. Pain with or without swelling
    B. Symptomless mass in extremity
    C. Edema in extremity
    D. Neuropathy in hands or feet

43. Radiographs may show a blastic or lytic tumor. Which of the following does not accurately describe the lesions:

    A. Blastic lesions project white on radiographs
    B. Blastic lesions are tumors where abnormal bone has built up onto normal bone
    C. Lytic lesions appear black on radiographs
    D. Lytic lesions are tumors where abnormal bone has built up onto normal bone

44. What diagnostic procedure is not commonly part of a patient's work-up if it is suspected that they may have a primary bone tumor?

    A. MRI
    B. Bone scan
    C. CEA tumor marking
    D. Biopsy

45. What histology of primary bone tumors is the most common?

    A. Fibrosarcoma
    B. Metastatic bone tumors
    C. Osteosarcoma
    D. Multiple myeloma

46. The most common location of osteosarcomas is:

    A. Diaphysis of long bones
    B. Metaphysis of flat bones
    C. Diaphysis of sesamoid bones
    D. Metaphysis of long bones

47. What type of recurrences are common in primary bone tumors?

    A. Local recurrence
    B. Distant spread to brain
    C. Lymphatic spread to para-aortic lymph nodes
    D. All of the above

48. Which treatment option is commonly used to treat primary bone cancer?

    A. Surgery and postoperative radiation therapy
    B. Concomitant chemo-RT
    C. Neo-adjuvant chemotherapy and surgery
    D. Radiation therapy alone

49. When treating bone tumors with external beam radiation therapy, which
    statement best describes the treatment?

    A. 30 Gy in 10 fx may be used for primary bone tumors
    B. IORT technique may be used
    C. The entire limb must be in the treatment field, including the scar and flashing
       on the lateral and medial aspect
    D. A and C
    E. B and C

50. Which of the following is not a late toxicity of external beam radiation therapy
    to the limb?

    A. Erythema
    B. Growth abnormalities
    C. Pathologic fractures
    D. Secondary malignancies

51. Soft tissue sarcomas are typically diagnosed in what decade of life?

    A. Third
    B. Fourth
    C. Fifth
    D. Sixth

52. Kaposi's sarcoma is linked to what virus?

    A. Epstein-Barr
    B. Human immunodeficiency virus
    C. Hepatitis C
    D. Human Papilloma

53. Soft tissue sarcomas can be caused by all of the following except:

   A. Genetics
   B. Radiation exposure
   C. Prior chemotherapy
   D. Trauma

54. What is the most common sign or symptom of soft tissue sarcomas?

   A. Pain in extremity, with or without swelling
   B. Painless mass
   C. Swelling in extremity
   D. Tingling sensation in digits

55. _____ is the most useful imaging exam to determine the size and location of soft tissue sarcomas.

   A. Chest radiograph
   B. CT
   C. PET
   D. MRI

56. The most common histology of soft tissue sarcomas in adults is:

   A. Liposarcoma
   B. Malignant fibrous histiocytoma
   C. Rhabdomyosarcoma
   D. Leiomyosarcoma

57. The most common histology of soft tissue sarcomas in children is:

   A. Liposarcoma
   B. Malignant fibrous histiocytoma
   C. Rhabdomyosarcoma
   D. Leiomyosarcoma

58. A sarcoma of the smooth muscle is:

   A. Liposarcoma
   B. Malignant fibrous histiocytoma
   C. Rhabdomyosarcoma
   D. Leiomyosarcoma

59. A sarcoma of adipose tissue is:

   A. Liposarcoma
   B. Malignant fibrous histiocytoma
   C. Rhabdomyosarcoma
   D. Leiomyosarcoma

60. Which of the following is true regarding the spread of soft tissue sarcomas?

    A. Local invasion is not common
    B. Distantly, soft tissue sarcomas spread to lungs, bone and liver
    C. Lymphatic spread is common
    D. All of the above are true

61. If treating soft tissue sarcoma with radiation therapy, what total dose would you use?

    A. 40–46 Gy
    B. 50–56 Gy
    C. 60–66 Gy
    D. 70–76 Gy

62. In addition to external beam radiation therapy, what other treatment may be used in the treatment of soft tissue sarcomas? Choose all correct answers.

    A. Surgery
    B. Brachytherapy
    C. Intrathecal chemotherapy
    D. IORT

63. Which of the following in not included when designing radiation therapy fields for soft tissue sarcomas?

    A. Scar
    B. Bolus
    C. Shrinking fields
    D. 1 cm margins

64. Ewing's sarcoma spreads distantly to the:

    A. Brain
    B. Liver
    C. Lungs
    D. Distant spread is rare

65. Radiographically, Ewing's sarcoma presents with:

    A. Onion skin appearance on periosteum
    B. Spiculated masses
    C. Abnormal Halversion canals
    D. Depleted bone marrow reserves

66. Which is true regarding Ewing's sarcoma? Choose all correct answers.

    A. Most common in children 4–10 years old
    B. Occurs equally in females and males
    C. Commonly found in extremities
    D. Presents with pain and swelling

67. Which statement is not true regarding pediatric medulloblastoma?

    A. Tumors are most commonly located in the frontal lobe
    B. Patients present with signs and symptoms of increased intracranial pressure
    C. CSF seeding is common
    D. Peak incidence is 5 years old

68. Which of the following accurately describes radiation therapy treatment of medulloblastoma?

    A. Entire craniospinal axis is treated to dose of 56 Gy.
    B. Treatment is to the primary tumor location only to a total dose of 56 Gy
    C. Patient blood counts must be monitored closely during treatment
    D. Radiation therapy is given preoperatively

69. Wilm's tumor is a pediatric tumor of the:

    A. Kidney
    B. Liver
    C. Spleen
    D. Adrenal gland

70. Patients with Wilm's tumor often present with:

    A. Back pain
    B. Jaundice
    C. Painless abdominal mass
    D. Increased ADCH production

71. When treating Wilm's disease, radiation therapists must ensure:

    A. Entire pelvis is in the treatment field
    B. Medial border includes the entire width of the spinal body
    C. The prescription has a total dose of 40 Gy
    D. The inferior border is placed inferior to the obturator foramen

72. Neuroblastoma is a malignancy of the:

    A. Kidney
    B. Liver
    C. Spleen
    D. Adrenal gland

73. Which of the following is true regarding neuroblastoma?

    A. Radiation therapy is the primary treatment modality
    B. Distant metastasis is rare
    C. Tumors may spontaneously regress
    D. Patients present with increased albumin levels

74. Leukocaria is a presenting sign of:

    A. Rhabdomyosarcoma
    B. Choroid melanoma
    C. Optic neuroma
    D. Retinoblastoma

75. Which of the following radiation therapy treatment is not used to treat retinoblastoma?

    A. Proton therapy
    B. Eye plaques
    C. External beam with lens block
    D. Opposed lateral electron beams

76. Which of the following is not a common site for rhabdomyosarcomas?

    A. Brain
    B. GU system
    C. Extremities
    D. Trunk

77. Pediatric brain tumors are (choose all correct answers):

    A. Intratentorial
    B. Least common solid tumor in pediatric patients
    C. Diagnosed with MRI and lumbar punctures

78. Heterotopic bone formation is treated with a total dose of:

    A. 7 Gy
    B. 15 Gy
    C. 21 Gy
    D. 28 Gy

Answers and Rationales

1. C. Exposure to ionizing radiation is a risk factor for developing leukemia.
   There are approximately 44,000 new cases of leukemia a year, 50 % acute and 50 % chronic. ALL is #1 leukemia in pediatric patients, between ages of 2 and 3, while AML is common in pts over the age of 40, median age 67. While the cause of leukemia is mostly unknown, genetic links and exposure to ionizing radiation are risk factors for developing leukemia.
2. A and C. In addition to petechiae and epitaxis, patients may also present with malaise and flu-like symptoms.
3. D. MRIs are not used routinely to diagnose leukemia, as leukemia does not form solid tumors.
4. A. CML stands for chronic myelogenous leukemia. ALL stands for acute lymphocytic leukemia, AML stands for acute myelogenous leukemia, and CLL stands for chronic lymphocytic leukemia.
5. B and C. Because leukemia spreads hematologoneously, chemotherapy is the primary treatment. Total-body irradiation and bone marrow transplants are also used.
6. A. Allogeneic transplants use bone marrow from a donor, while syngeneic transplants use bone marrow from a twin.
7. A, B, and E. While the patient position differs from facility to facility, patients are treated at an extended distance to the entire body. Lungs are blocked, and compensators are placed at the head and feet. Patients are treated twice a day at 300 cGy per fraction for a total dose of 1200 cGy. TLDs are placed on ankles, knees, and thighs. Patients are often in neutropenic precautions.
8. B. This field is treated to a total dose of 18 Gy.
9. D. The bimodal age distribution describes the peak of incidence in 25–30-year-olds (most common) and 75–80-year-olds.
10. B. The Epstein-Barr virus in linked to Hodgkin's disease.
11. C. One-third of patients present with B symptoms (night sweats, fever, and weight loss). Patients most commonly present with a painless mass in the neck.
12. B. There are four subtypes of Hodgkin's disease. Nodular sclerosing is the most common. Other types include mixed cellularity, lymphocytic predominant (most radiosensitive) and lymphocytic depleted (worst prognosis).
13. B. Presence of the Reed Sternberg cell indicates a diagnosis of Hodgkin's disease.
14. A. The Ann Arbor staging system is used to stage Hodgkin's disease.
15. B. Hodgkin's disease spreads through lymph node groups in a contiguous fashion.
16. B. Treatment for Hodgkin's disease may include MOPP or AVBD chemotherapy, or radiation therapy to the involved nodes.
17. C. Mantle fields are used to treat lymph nodes above diaphragm, with AP/PA fields. The superior border is placed inferior to the mandible, while the inferior border is placed at T10. The field is wide enough to include the axilla.
18. A and D. The organs at risk in a tradition mantle field include humeral heads, lung, heart, spinal cord, larynx, thyroid, and esophagus. Acute toxicities are

myelosuppression, fatigue, and dysphagia, while late toxicities patients may experience include radiation pneumonitis, secondary malignancies, hypothyroidism, and cardiovascular disease.

19. A. Inverted Y fields treat lymph nodes below diaphragm with AP/PA fields to a dose of 20–36 Gy. The superior border matches that of the mantle field and is placed at T10. The inferior border is placed 2 cm below the ischial tuberosity (split at L4/L5). The fields are 8–10 cm wide, centered on lymph nodes. Testicular shields are used for men, while women may have an oophoropexy prior to treatment.

20. A, B, and C. Organs at risk for Inverted Y fields include the kidneys, liver, ovaries, and testes. Acute toxicities include myelosuppression, nausea and vomiting, diarrhea, and cystitis, while late toxicities may include fertility problems and secondary malignancies.

21. C. There are approximately 66,000 new cases of non-Hodgkin's lymphoma each year. The average age at diagnosis is 65 years of age. Risk factors for non-Hodgkin's lymphoma include Burkitt's lymphoma, Epstein-Barr virus, occupational and environmental exposures, and exposure to ionizing radiation.

22. D. Spread of non-Hodgkin's lymphoma is noncontiguous, and commonly spread to extranodal sites (spleen, CNS, GI, Waldeyer's ring).

23. A. Chemotherapy is the primary treatment for non-Hodgkin's lymphoma, specifically CHOP and R-CHOP chemotherapy agents.

24. B. Thyroid cancer is the most prevalent cancer of the endocrine system. It occurs more often in females, and is linked to radiation exposure. Patients may present with swelling of the neck, hoarseness and difficulty swallowing.

25. A. Diagnostic exams used to diagnose thyroid cancer include labs to check thyroid function, ultrasound, iodine imaging, and FNA biopsy.

26. A. Papillary, mixed papillar-follicular is the most common, while anaplastic histology is very aggressive. Other types of thyroid cancer include follicular and medullary histology.

27. C. Anaplastic thyroid cancer typically spreads through local invasion into surrounding structures, while papillary thyroid cancer spreads through the lymphatic system. Follicular thyroid cancer spreads distantly to the bone, lung, liver, and brain.

28. C. In addition to surgery, I-131 ablation is a common treatment for thyroid cancer.

29. D. Pituitary tumors are usually benign tumors. Common presentations include hormonal changes, headaches, and visual changes. Work-up for pituitary tumors includes MRI and lab work to check hormone levels.

30. B. Treatments for pituitary tumors include surgery (transphenoidal hypophysectomy) or radiation therapy. Radiation therapy may be delivered through arc treatments or IMRT to a total dose of 45–50.4 Gy, or SRS to a total dose of 15–25 Gy.

31. A, C, and D. Organs at risk for pituitary cancers include the optic nerve, optic chiasm, brain, ear, and lens.

32. D. Skin cancer is the most common malignancy in the US, with over one million new cases diagnosed each year.

33. A, B, and D. Risk factors for skin cancer include UV exposure, having a fair complexion or prior skin cancer.

34. C. Common signs or symptoms of skin cancer include ABCD (asymmetry, irregular borders, irregular color, and increasing diameter) and sores that do not heal.

35. A. Melanoma skin cancers have the propensity to spread, so a complete work-up is needed.

36. C. Basal cell carcinomas are the most common histology of skin cancer.

37. A. Treatment for melanoma is surgery, with or without chemotherapy and immunotherapy. Nonmelanoma skin cancers are treated with surgery (Moh's technique), radiation therapy, or topical chemotherapy.

38. A. Moh's surgery involves taking layer by layer of skin until no tumor is present. This surgery is commonly used in the treatment of skin cancer and provides better cosmetic results.

39. B. Single electron fields or orthovoltage photons may be used to treat skins cancers, with a margin of 1–2 cm around the lesion. Fields are treated to a total dose of 50–60 Gy, and bolus may be utilized.

40. B. Erythema, dry desquamation, moist desquamation and alopecia are acute toxicities of radiation therapy to the skin. Late toxicities include fibrosis and permanent skin changes.

41. B and D. Primary bone tumors are rare, with approximately 2400 cases diagnosed each year. This type of cancer is more common in males, and patients less than 35 years old. There is a genetic link to some subtypes, and a history of Paget's disease or radiation exposure increases the risk of developing primary bone cancer.

42. A. Most primary bone tumors present with pain in the bone, with or without swelling.

43. D. Lytic lesions show up black on radiographs, indicating where bone has been eaten away, while blastic lesions show up white on radiographs.

44. C. Diagnostic procedures include radiographs, MRI, bone scans, and biopsies.

45. C. While metastatic bone tumors are the most common tumor in the bone, osteosarcoma is the most common histology of primary bone tumors.

46. D. The most common location of osteosarcomas is the metaphysis of long bones, especially distal femur, proximal tibia, and proximal humerus.

47. A. Primary bone tumors recur locally. Osteosarcoma may spread distantly to the lung.

48. C. Neoadjuvant chemotherapy and surgery is used for the treatment of primary bone tumors. Radiation therapy is not commonly used for primary bone tissues due to radioresistancy of tumors.

49. B. 30 Gy in 10 fx may be used for metastatic bone tumors, but high doses are needed for primary bone tumors. IORT may be used, and if EBRT is used the field should include scar as well as preserve a strip of skin to preserve lymphatics.

50. A. Erythema is an acute toxicity.

51. C. Soft tissue sarcomas are rare, with only 10,000 cases diagnosed per year. They are commonly diagnosed in patients between ages of 40 and 50 years old.

52. B. Kaposi's sarcoma is linked to Human immunodeficiency virus.

53. D. Trauma is not a risk factor for development of soft tissue sarcomas.
54. B. A painless mass in an extremity is the most common presentation of soft tissue sarcomas. Pain and numbness are other symptoms of soft tissue sarcomas.
55. D. MRI is the primary diagnostic exam for soft tissue sarcomas, but PET, CT, and chest radiographs may also be used in the work up.
56. B. Malignant fibrous histiocytoma is the most common soft tissue sarcoma in adults.
57. C. Rhabdomyosarcoma (sarcoma of skeletal muscles) is the most common sarcoma in pediatric patients.
58. D. Leiomyosarcoma is a sarcoma of smooth muscle.
59. A. Liposarcoma is a sarcoma of adipose tissue.
60. B. Local invasion is common with soft tissue sarcomas. These tumors also spread distantly to the lungs, bone, and liver. Lymphatic spread is not common.
61. C. Doses of 60–66 Gy are used to treat soft tissue sarcomas.
62. A, B, and D. Surgery ± radiation therapist and chemotherapy is used in the treatment of soft tissue sarcomas. Radiation therapy may be in the form of EBRT, IORT, or brachytherapy.
63. D. Fields should include the scar (may need bolus), use wide (5 cm) margins around GTV, and a shrinking field technique may be used.
64. C. Ewing's sarcoma also spreads locally. Lung metastasis may be treated with whole lung radiation therapy fields to total dose of 15 Gy.
65. A. Radiographically, Ewing's sarcoma has an onion-skin appearance of the periosteum.
66. C and D. Ewing's sarcoma peaks in patients ages 10–20 years old, and is more common in males than females. These tumors are more likely to occur in extremities, especially the femur.
67. A. Medulloblastoma tumors are an infratentorial brain tumor.
68. C. Primary treatment for medulloblastoma is surgery, followed by craniospinal irradiation to a dose of 25–36 Gy with a boost to the posterior fossa to 56 Gy. Due to the large amount of bone marrow in the treatment fields, blood counts must be monitored closely during treatment.
69. A. Wilm's tumor is a pediatric tumor of the kidney (nephroblastoma).
70. C. Patients with Wilm's tumor often present with a painless abdominal mass.
71. B. The radiation therapist must ensure the medial border includes the entire spinal body to prevent scoliosis.
72. D. Neuroblastomas occur in the adrenal glands.
73. C. Patients with neuroblastoma are often lethargic and present with an abdominal mass. Surgery is primary treatment, but the tumors can spontaneously regress.
74. D. Retinoblastoma can present with leukocoria and/or strabismus.
75. D. Along with enoculation, radiation therapy may be used for the treatment of retinoblastoma. Radiation therapy can be delivered with external photon beams, eye plaques or proton therapy.
76. A. Rhabdomyosarcomas are the most common soft tissue sarcoma in pediatric patients. They commonly occur in the head and neck, GU, extremities and trunk.

77. A and C. Pediatric brain tumors are intratentorial, and the most common solid tumor in pediatric patients. These tumors are diagnosed with MRI and lumbar punctures.
78. A. A single treatment of 7 Gy is adequate to stop the overgrowth process.

Suggested Readings

Adams RD, Newell T. Endocrine system tumors. In: Washington CM, Leaver D, editors. Principles and practice of radiation therapy. 3rd ed. St. Louis, MO: Mosby Elsevier; 2010. p. 643–65.

Bartenhagen L, Koth J. Bone, cartilage and soft tissue sarcomas. In: Washington CM, Leaver D, editors. Principles and practice of radiation therapy. 3rd ed. St. Louis, MO: Mosby Elsevier; 2010. p. 581–609.

Belinsky SB, McKenney MA. Leukemia. In: Washington CM, Leaver D, editors. Principles and practice of radiation therapy. 3rd ed. St. Louis, MO: Mosby Elsevier; 2010. p. 628–42.

Burri RJ. Thyroid. In: Chao KSC, Perez CA, Brady LW, editors. Radiation oncology management decisions. 3rd ed. Philadelphia, PA: Wolters Kluwer-Lippincott Williams and Wilkins; 2011. p. 319–26.

Deutsch I. Skin cancer, acquired immunodeficiency syndrome related malignancies, and Kaposi's sarcoma. In: Chao KSC, Perez CA, Brady LW, editors. Radiation oncology management decisions. 3rd ed. Philadelphia, PA: Wolters Kluwer-Lippincott Williams and Wilkins; 2011. p. 119–34.

Green S. Lymphoreticular system tumors. In: Washington CM, Leaver D, editors. Principles and practice of radiation therapy. 3rd ed. St. Louis, MO: Mosby Elsevier; 2010. p. 610–27.

Lewis VO. The bone. In: Cox JD, Ang KK, editors. Radiation oncology: rationale, treatment, results. 9th ed. St. Louis, MO: Mosby Elsevier; 2009. p. 915–39.

Sheplan LJ, Macklis RM. Lymphoma and myeloma radiotherapy. In: Videtic GMM, Vassil AD, editors. Handbook of treatment planning in radiation oncology. New York: Demos Medical Publishing; 2011. p. 158–80.

Vance WZ, Shah AA. Hodgkin's disease. In: Chao KSC, Perez CA, Brady LW, editors. Radiation oncology management decisions. 3rd ed. Philadelphia, PA: Wolters Kluwer-Lippincott Williams and Wilkins; 2011a. p. 639–58.

Vance WZ, Shah AA. Non-Hodgkin's lymphoma. In: Chao KSC, Perez CA, Brady LW, editors. Radiation oncology management decisions. 3rd ed. Philadelphia, PA: Wolters Kluwer-Lippincott Williams and Wilkins; 2011b. p. 659–80.

Vann A, Dasher BG, Wiggers NH, Chesnut SK. Portal design in radiation therapy. 3rd ed. Augusta, GA: DWV Enterprises; 2013.

Washington CM. Skin cancers and melanoma. In: Washington CM, Leaver D, editors. Principles and practice of radiation therapy. 3rd ed. St. Louis, MO: Mosby Elsevier; 2010. p. 912–37.

Wuu CS, Marinetti T. Advanced treatment technology (IMRT, SRS, SBRT, IGRT, Proton Beam Therapy). In: Chao KSC, Perez CA, Brady LW, editors. Radiation oncology management decisions. 3rd ed. Philadelphia, PA: Wolters Kluwer-Lippincott Williams and Wilkins; 2011. p. 41–56.

Young J. Pediatric solid tumors. In: Washington CM, Leaver D, editors. Principles and practice of radiation therapy. 3rd ed. St. Louis, MO: Mosby Elsevier; 2010. p. 895–911.

Index

© Springer Science+Business Media New York 2016
A. Heath, *Radiation Therapy Study Guide*, DOI 10.1007/978-1-4939-3258-0

Printed in the United States
By Bookmasters